Dr. Mark Stengler's Natural Healing Library

- Foods That Heal

- Natural Cures That Work Better Than Drugs

- New Breakthroughs in Holistic Medicine

- Free Cures and Low-Cost Home Remedies

- Help or Hype? The Truth About What Works and What Doesn't

- Hidden Health Dangers: What You Don't Know Can Hurt You

- How to Spot Health Problems Early By Reading Your Body's Hidden Signals

- No-Willpower Weight Loss

- How to Find a Good Holistic Doctor in Your Area

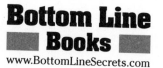

Bottom Line Books

www.BottomLineSecrets.com

Contents

SPECIAL REPORT #7:

HOW TO SPOT HEALTH PROBLEMS EARLY BY READING YOUR BODY'S HIDDEN SIGNALS

SPECIAL REPORT #8:

NO-WILLPOWER WEIGHT LOSS

SPECIAL REPORT #9:

HOW TO FIND A GOOD HOLISTIC DOCTOR IN YOUR AREA

SPECIAL REPORT #1:

Foods That Heal

Foods That Heal

Seven Super Foods— Delicious Ways to Fight Disease

Nearly 2,500 years ago, Hippocrates, the father of modern medicine, said, *"Let food be thy medicine and medicine be thy food."* This is still true today—the right foods help you stay healthy and are powerful disease fighters. *Here are seven of the best...*

1. Beans

Americans' consumption of beans has steadily increased over the past two decades, and that's good news because beans have tremendous healing power. Popular varieties include soybeans, garbanzo (chickpeas), pinto, kidney, lima, navy and black beans. Beans are a type of legume, a class of vegetable that also includes lentils and peas.

Beans are high in protein, low in fat and calories, and rich in complex carbohydrates, fiber, phytonutrients and several vitamins and minerals, including folic acid and other B vitamins, potassium, magnesium and iron.

In addition, beans are loaded with soluble fiber, the same type of gummy fiber found in the oat bran in oatmeal. This type of fiber helps bind and eliminate cholesterol and stabilize blood sugar levels.

A study conducted by the US Department of Agriculture found that beans—especially black, pinto and kidney beans—topped the list of vegetables that are rich in disease-fighting antioxidants.

Specifically, several studies have shown that regular consumption of beans significantly reduces the risk for cardiovascular disease. New studies are now suggesting that beans also have potent anticancer properties. Both meat eaters and vegetarians enjoy this easy-to-find food.

Mark A. Stengler, ND, naturopathic physician in private practice, La Jolla, California...adjunct associate clinical professor at the National College of Natural Medicine, Portland, Oregon...author of many books, including *The Natural Physician's Healing Therapies* and coauthor of *Prescription for Natural Cures* (both from Bottom Line Books)...and author of the *Bottom Line/Natural Healing* newsletter.

Recommended: Eat one-half cup of beans four times weekly. Beans make an excellent addition to salads, rice dishes and soups, and they can be pureed as a dip.

Helpful: Many people avoid beans because they experience gas after eating them. If this is a problem, take an enzyme product such as Beano, available at most grocery stores and drugstores. Follow directions on the label.

2. Broccoli

I am thankful that broccoli is such a popular food in my household—all three of my children like it. This king of the cruciferous family (other members include brussels sprouts, cabbage, kale, cauliflower and bok choy) is an excellent source of vitamin C, vitamin A, folic acid, calcium and fiber.

Broccoli fights cancer. It contains two classes of anticancer phytonutrients—*isothiocyanates* and *glucosinolates.*

•*Sulforaphane* is an isothiocyanate that activates detoxifying enzymes in the body that prevent the formation of cancer-causing substances. Sulforaphane also has potent antioxidant properties.

•*Indole-3-carbinol* (I3C) is a glucosinolate that has been shown to benefit women with early-stage cervical cancer and helps protect estrogen-sensitive cells, such as breast cells.

Broccoli also is rich in the carotenoid antioxidants *lutein* and *zeaxanthin*. Both are important in preventing ultraviolet damage to the eyes and can help prevent cataracts and age-related macular degeneration, the leading cause of blindness in people age 65 and older.

Recommended: Eat one-half cup of raw or lightly steamed broccoli daily (buying frozen broccoli is fine). Avoid boiling—it diminishes its nutritional value.

Broccoli sprouts, which are the newly sprouted seeds of broccoli, can be added to sandwiches or salads. They contain 30 to 50 times the concentration of protective phytonutrients that are found in mature broccoli plants. Broccoli sprouts are especially rich in sulforaphane. Because broccoli sprouts can be contaminated with bacteria, people with weak immune systems should check with their doctors before consuming them.

3. Eggs

The egg is an excellent source of protein, and it contains all the essential amino acids that your body cannot produce on its own. In addition, it is a rich source of vitamin K, cancer-fighting selenium, vitamin B-12 and choline, a nutrient required by cell membranes for healthy function. Some of these nutrients are found in the yolk, so egg whites alone are not as beneficial.

In the past, the egg got a bad reputation when it came to cholesterol and heart disease. However, multiple studies have now vindicated the egg.

A study in the *Journal of the American Medical Association*, conducted at Harvard School of Public Health, found no relationship between egg consumption and cardiovascular disease in a population of more than 117,000 nurses and health professionals who were followed for eight to 14 years. There was no difference in heart disease risk between those who ate less than one egg a week and those who ate one egg a day.

In fact, the protein in eggs appears to prevent blood clots. Eggs also contain the eye-protective nutrient lutein—and lutein from eggs is more easily absorbed than that from spinach (one of the richest sources) or from supplements.

In addition, in one Chinese study, women who ate at least six eggs a week lowered their risk of breast cancer by 44%, compared with no risk reduction in women who consumed two or fewer eggs a week.

Recommended: Eat one to six organic eggs weekly. Organic eggs don't contain hormone or antibiotic residues.

Caution: People with gallbladder disease should avoid eggs. Eggs may worsen symptoms, including pain and spasms, possibly due to the fat content.

4. Blueberries

One of nature's antiaging stars, blueberries contain a megasupply of powerful antioxidants known as *anthocyanins*, which help protect against cell damage. Anthocyanins have been shown to enhance the effects of vitamin C, improve capillaries so they're less likely to rupture and support the body's connective tissues. Anthocyanins give blueberries their blue-purple color. Blueberries also are a good source of vitamin C and vitamin E, manganese and fiber.

Blueberries contain the anthocyanin *pterostilbene*, a powerful antioxidant compound that is known to fight cancer. Animal studies have shown that pterostilbene also reduces cholesterol, improves memory and shortens recovery time from stroke. In addition, blueberries promote good eye health—they are particularly helpful in the prevention of macular degeneration.

Like cranberries, blueberries have been found to contain substances that prevent bacteria from adhering to the lining of the urinary tract, which may help guard against urinary tract infections.

Recommended: Eat one-half cup of blueberries five times weekly. Sprinkle blueberries, fresh or frozen, on cereal or add them to muffins and smoothies.

5. Oatmeal

Oatmeal, one of the most nutritious complex carbohydrates, contains several vital minerals, including manganese, selenium, magnesium, zinc and copper.

Oatmeal also provides protein and, as I mentioned earlier, is an excellent source of soluble fiber. Because this type of fiber stabilizes blood sugar, oatmeal is an excellent choice for people with diabetes.

The best-known benefits of this super food are its cholesterol-lowering properties. A type of soluble fiber known as *beta-glucan* (which also activates immune cells) and compounds called *saponins* bind dietary cholesterol and usher it out of the body unabsorbed.

A daily bowl of oatmeal can reduce total cholesterol by as much as 23%. It has also been shown to reduce the "bad" LDL cholesterol without changing levels of beneficial HDL cholesterol.

In addition, oats are a rich source of *tocotrienols*. These relatives of the vitamin E family guard against the oxidation of LDL cholesterol (thereby preventing LDL cholesterol from sticking to artery walls and causing plaque buildup) and reduce the production of cholesterol by the liver.

Recommended: Eat one cup of oatmeal three to four times weekly. When possible, choose the longer-cooking variety—instant oatmeal has a weaker cholesterol-lowering effect and often has salt and sugar added. Oatmeal is even healthier when sprinkled with a tablespoon of ground flaxseed and one-half teaspoon of cinnamon, both of which help lower cholesterol.

6. Walnuts

Walnuts are the perfect snack. They are rich in omega-3 fatty acids, which reduce inflammation in the body. Walnuts also contain the minerals manganese and copper, both of which play key roles in the body's antioxidant network.

In addition, these tasty nuts contain *gamma-tocopherol*, a component of vitamin E that provides antioxidant protection, as well as the amino acid *l-arginine*, which improves circulation. Walnuts also contain the phytonutrient *ellagic acid*, which helps protect against cancer-causing free radical damage.

Walnuts also are a source of the sleep hormone *melatonin*. The amount is too small to promote sleep, but the melatonin in walnuts provides additional antioxidant activity.

Several studies have shown that the consumption of walnuts reduces the risk of coronary artery disease. One study found that a walnut-rich diet lowered levels of *C-reactive protein*, a marker of inflammation, which is strongly associated with atherosclerosis and heart disease. Walnuts not only increase levels of omega-3 fatty acids but also decrease the adhesion of cholesterol to the lining of the arteries.

A study conducted at the Lipid Clinic at the Endocrinology and Nutrition Service, Institut d'Investigacions Biomediques in Barcelona, Spain, showed that a walnut-rich diet reduced total cholesterol by 4.4% and LDL cholesterol by 6.4%.

Other studies have found that walnuts significantly increase the elasticity of the arteries, which is a marker for healthy blood vessels. The Food and Drug Administration allows walnuts to carry the health claim that "eating 1.5 ounces of walnuts per day as part of a diet low in saturated fat and cholesterol may reduce the risk for heart disease."

Recommended: Eat four to eight walnuts (approximately 1.5 ounces) daily in cereals, salads and yogurt—or eat them plain.

7. Yogurt

Yogurt is a fermented dairy product rich in "friendly" bacteria. These bacteria, such as *Lactobacillus acidophilus* and *Lactobacillus bulgaricus*, improve immune function. Yogurt also is a good source of calcium, phosphorus, vitamin B-2 (riboflavin), iodine, vitamin B-12, vitamin B-5 (pantothenic acid), zinc, potassium and protein. Several studies have shown that incorporating calcium-rich foods, such as low-fat yogurt and cheese, into a reduced-calorie diet is an effective weight-management technique.

Yogurt also suppresses the growth of *Helicobacter pylori*, the bacterium that causes most cases of stomach ulcer. Along with other dairy products, yogurt appears to protect against colon and rectal cancers—perhaps because of the calcium content. Studies also have found that yogurt reduces the compounds that contribute to bad breath, cavities and gum disease.

Recommended: Eat one-half to one cup of yogurt daily. Look for low-fat yogurts that list "live active cultures" or "living yogurt cultures" on the label.

Do not buy any yogurt that contains artificial color, flavoring or sweetener. Choose plain yogurt or flavored yogurt made by Horizon or other companies that don't use artificial ingredients. Opt for organic yogurt products to avoid hormone and antibiotic residues. Yogurt is delicious when used in place of milk in cereals or as part of a smoothie.

Caution: Avoid yogurt if you are allergic or sensitive to cow's milk—goat's milk yogurt is an option.

The Truth About Brain Food...and Supplements That Keep Your Memory Intact

Everyone forgets something from time to time. Some people have trouble remembering names. Others can't keep track of their car keys. Whether we suffer everyday absentmindedness or moments of real memory loss, all of us are concerned about keeping our brain power intact.

In recent years, a great deal of research has focused on the most severe kinds of memory loss—senile dementia and Alzheimer's disease.

In the US, these closely related conditions affect up to 10% of people over age 65 and nearly half of those over age 85.

Many studies have identified ways to lower risk of these age-related problems. Popular methods include stress-reduction strategies, such as daily exercise, positive mental imagery, biofeedback and close personal relationships, to prevent spikes in the memory-draining stress hormone *cortisol*..."brain workouts," including crossword puzzles, word games and challenging card games...and eight to nine hours of sleep each night. Good nutrition—and the right kind of supplementation—also can help protect our brains and safeguard our memories at any age. The sooner you get started with a brain-protecting regimen, the more you'll benefit.

For optimal brain function, your diet should be well-balanced with carbohydrates (40%), protein (30%) and fats (30%). You can accomplish this by eating meals that include whole grains, fruits and vegetables (for complex carbohydrates)...fish, poultry, lean meats, legumes, nuts and seeds (for protein)...and fish oil, olive oil, avocados, almonds, walnuts and ground flaxseed (for fats). Steer clear of dairy products and packaged and processed foods, such as cookies, white bread and pasta, which are packed with simple carbohydrates that wreak havoc on glucose levels, contributing to diabetes, stroke/vascular disease and dementia.

THE VALUE OF FISH

Fish provides *docosahexaenoic acid* (DHA) and *eicosapentaenoic acid* (EPA), the most plentiful fatty acids in the brain. DHA, an omega-3 fatty acid, is found in abundance in cold-water fish such as mackerel, sardines, salmon and herring. You also can get it from fish-oil supplements, egg yolks, DHA-enriched eggs and some algae supplements, such as Neuromins, a product that is available at most health-food stores. Foods such as walnuts...leafy, green vegetables...and supplements including flaxseed and hemp oil contain *alpha-linolenic acid*, an omega-3 fatty acid that can be converted by the body into DHA and EPA.

How essential is DHA to memory? It has been known for some years that people have a higher risk of Alzheimer's if they have low blood levels of DHA. A study in *Archives of Neurology* revealed

6

that people who ate fish one to three times a month had a 40% lower risk of Alzheimer's than those who never ate fish. Those who consumed fish once a week or more had a 60% lower risk. Fish may be baked, broiled or grilled.

It also makes sense to take a fish-oil supplement daily. I suggest 1,000 mg of combined DHA and EPA. Good brands are Nordic Naturals (800-622-2544, *www.nordicnaturals.com*) and Carlson Laboratories (888-234-5656, *www.carlsonlabs.com*), both available at health-food stores. Caution: Fish oil can thin blood, so check with your doctor before using it if you take blood-thinning medications such as *warfarin* (Coumadin).

GLA IS ESSENTIAL

Omega-6s make up another class of essential fatty acids that are necessary for good brain function. Omega-6 is found in vegetable oils, including safflower, sunflower and corn oils. Most American diets contain too much of these oils due to consumption of packaged and fried foods. However, the most important omega-6 fatty acid is *linoleic acid*, which is converted in the body to *gamma-linolenic acid* (GLA). This essential fatty acid plays a big role in the formation of healthy brain-cell membranes, the part of the cell that stores information. Taking borage oil or evening primrose oil is a healthful way to increase GLA intake—hempseed and hempseed oil also are good sources. Another way to get GLA in the diet is by consuming flaxseed (with water to prevent constipation) or flaxseed oil.

COUNT ON CHOLINE

Just as a car needs spark plugs, an active brain needs quick-firing neurotransmitters. As the name implies, a neurotransmitter sends a signal that jumps from one brain cell to another. Substances that act as neurotransmitters—the most important of which is a brain chemical called *acetylcholine*—are vital components of the brain's communication system.

There's one hitch. In order for your body to manufacture enough *acetylcholine*, you need to get a closely related nutrient called *choline*. The best source of choline is *phosphatidylcholine* (PC), which occurs naturally in fish, egg yolks, legumes, nuts, meat and vegetables. It also is found in breast milk. To help prevent memory

problems, you can boost your PC intake by taking a 1,500-mg to 2,000-mg PC supplement daily. (Doses of more than 3,000 mg can cause digestive upset, including diarrhea, nausea and stomachache.)

PC is only part of the neurotransmitter equation. To turn PC into brain-friendly *choline*, you also need to get healthy doses of vitamin C and certain B vitamins. You can get plenty of these vitamins in your diet by eating red, yellow and green peppers, citrus fruits and cantaloupe for vitamin C and sweet potatoes, tuna and avocados for B vitamins. Also, I recommend taking a balanced daily multivitamin/mineral supplement.

Deficiencies of folic acid and other key B vitamins have been associated with an increased risk of Alzheimer's disease. These nutrients help to lower levels of *homocysteine*, a harmful byproduct of protein metabolism that is increased in people who are genetically susceptible. That's why it is important to have your blood levels of homocysteine, folic acid and B-12 tested by your doctor to see if you need additional supplementation of folic acid and/or B-12.

THE EUROPEAN CURE

For years, European doctors have recommended a supplement called *L-alpha-glycerylphosphorylcholine* (GPC) to promote mental acuity (the ability to respond quickly and appropriately to mental challenges). GPC actually is used by the brain more effectively than PC to form *acetylcholine*—but it costs twice as much and is less widely available in the US. A good GPC supplement by Source Naturals is sold in some health-food stores under the brand name Alpha GPC (to find a retailer, go to *www.sourcenaturals.com*). Take two 300-mg capsules twice daily for the first four weeks, then two 300-mg capsules once daily as a maintenance dosage. Side effects are rare, but take GPC with a meal if it seems to interfere with your digestion.

PS: BE SURE TO GET MORE

Phosphatidylserine (PS) is a fat that the brain needs to preserve the key brain chemicals *serotonin* and *dopamine*. It also has been shown to reduce levels of the stress hormone cortisol. PS is found in fish, soy and leafy, green vegetables. As we age, PS levels in the body start to decline, so most people need to take a supplement once they're past age 50.

A normal daily diet has about 70 mg of PS. You need about four times that much if you have memory problems. Nearly anyone can benefit from a 300-mg daily supplement of PS. You're likely to notice improvements in mental alertness after four to eight weeks. A small percentage of people have digestive upset, such as bloating and diarrhea, but you can reduce the dosage if this is a problem. PS is available at health-food stores and pharmacies. Make sure you buy a product that lists "phosphatidylserine" on the label. (Some supplements contain "phosphorylated serine," a nutrient complex that doesn't provide the same benefits as PS.) A high-quality PS supplement is made by Jarrow Formulas (to find a retailer, call 800-726-0886 or go to *www.jarrow.com*).

HELP FROM ALC

When taken as a supplement, a nutrient known as *acetyl-L-carnitine* (ALC) has been shown to improve cognitive function and memory in older adults. Researchers also have found that ALC slows the progression of early-stage Alzheimer's disease. By improving communication between the two main hemispheres of the brain, ALC helps enhance the interplay of creative and cognitive brain activity.

For people with mild memory problems, I recommend taking 500 mg of ALC daily on an empty stomach. For those with more severe problems such as dementia, I suggest the same dose three times daily. Cut back if you have digestive upset. Most health-food stores carry a reliable ALC formula produced by Now Foods (888-669-3663, *www.nowfoods.com*).

ADD ANTIOXIDANTS

In all likelihood, Alzheimer's disease and other types of dementia are related to excessive damage by free radicals (normal by-products of metabolism that can destroy cells, organs and tissues). Free radicals irreversibly injure our cells and contribute to accelerated aging, but studies have shown that this damage can be warded off by getting enough antioxidant nutrients to help guard our brain-cell membranes.

There's ample evidence that a daily dose of 2,000 international units (IU) of the powerful antioxidant vitamin E can slow the decline of cognitive function in people who have moderate to severe Alzheimer's disease. There have been controversial vitamin E studies that seemed to show a link to worsening chronic disease. However, I don't have much confidence in those studies because they were performed on unhealthy people. When it comes to Alzheimer's, results of vitamin E studies have been quite good.

All fresh fruits, vegetables and other plant foods provide multiple naturally occurring antioxidants. Juices are an especially concentrated source of antioxidants. In fact, a study of nearly 2,000 Japanese Americans found that those who reported drinking fruit and vegetable juices at least three times a week had a 75% lower risk of developing dementia than those who drank juices less than once a week. The most nutritious fruit juices include cranberry, pomegranate, apple and blueberry. I also like mixed vegetable juices containing any combination of spinach, celery, lettuce, parsley, watercress, carrot and tomato.

If there is a strong family history of dementia or you have beginning signs of it, take up to 2,000 IU of vitamin E daily. Green tea also is an excellent source of antioxidants. I recommend drinking two to four cups of green tea daily and eight ounces of fresh juice.

GINKGO—THE BRAIN PLEASER

Ginkgo biloba is an herbal remedy that has been shown to improve memory and cognitive processing by promoting blood flow to the brain. I recommend a 24% *flavoglycoside* extract. Start with a dose of 120 mg to 240 mg daily, and increase to 360 mg daily over a four-week period. Some people begin to see results in four to eight weeks. If you're already taking a blood-thinning medication such as aspirin or *warfarin*, consult your doctor before taking ginkgo.

Grocery Cart Smarts— What to Buy…and Why

Friends sometimes tease my wife, Angela, and me for being health-food fanatics, feigning amazement at our "exotic" meals. But then they ask, in all seriousness, for hands-on instruction in healthful food shopping. Going to the market with our family of five—including Angela (who is also a naturopathic doctor) and our three children, ages nine, six and four—they marvel at how much our kids know about nutrition.

That's why I thought it would be fun to take readers shopping, too. So come along for a tour of the market.

VERY HEALTHFUL VEGGIES

The fresher the food, the more nutritious it generally is, so we shop several times each week. We go to a nearby health-food store for locally grown produce (which hasn't spent days in transit) and organic products (which aren't contaminated with pesticides) and head straight for the vegetables.

●**Eggplant,** which Angela adores, is often the first item in our cart. The skin is a rich source of *nasunin*, a potent antioxidant (a substance that neutralizes disease-causing molecules called free radicals). Eggplant provides minerals that promote good circulation and/or strong bones, including potassium, manganese, copper and magnesium...plus B vitamins for heart health, including B-1 (thiamine), B-3 (niacin), B-6 (pyridoxine) and B-9 (folate). This versatile vegetable can be diced and stir-fried...thin-sliced and grilled...or cut in half, oven-baked until tender (about 20 minutes at 350 degrees), then topped with cottage cheese.

Note: Avoid eggplant if its *alkaloids* (organic compounds) aggravate your arthritis.

●**Beets** help to detoxify the body by raising levels of the antioxidant *glutathione* in the liver...improve gallbladder function by thinning bile (a digestive fluid)...and provide folate and manganese for joint health. Red beets provide the most *betacyanin*, a plant pigment that protects against colon cancer. Beets can be combined with carrots and juiced...grated and added to salads...or cut into chunks and roasted.

●**Broccoli** contains the antioxidants *sulforaphane* and *chlorophyl*...vitamins A, C and E, which strengthen the immune system...calcium and vitamin K for bone health...folate for normal cell division...and *lutein* (a plant pigment) for eye health. Cauliflower provides many of the same *phytonutrients* (beneficial plant chemicals) as broccoli.

●**Carrots** pack easily into lunch boxes. We love baby carrots dipped in salad dressing, so we buy dressings with no unhealthful hydrogenated fat, high-fructose corn syrup or *monosodium glutamate* (MSG), a salty additive. For carrot juice, we peel large carrots and put them in our Vita-Mix (from $449, 800-848-2649, *www.vita mix.com*), a high-power blender that preserves the fiber-rich pulp of fruits and vegetables.

●**Cabbage** is a super source of vitamin K (for bone health)...vitamin C (for tissue growth and repair)...and organic compounds called *indoles* (for cancer prevention). Red cabbage has more healthful plant pigments than white. Since its juice has a very mild flavor, Angela adds red cabbage to almost everything we make in the Vita-Mix. Our kids get a kick from the looks on their friends' faces when we add cabbage to a fruit sorbet or fruit smoothie—and it's even more fun when their friends love the taste!

●**Cherry tomatoes,** rich in vitamins A and C, taste great with sliced low-fat mozzarella cheese.

●**Salad greens** we eat daily include romaine, red- or green-leaf lettuce and fresh spinach. They provide vitamin K, as well as fiber for bowel regularity.

FAVORITE FRUITS

We love fresh fruit for snacks and desserts.

●**Mango,** one of my favorites, is rich in fiber, beta-carotene, magnesium, potassium and vitamins B-1, B-2 (riboflavin), B-3 and B-6. Sweet, tangy and juicy, mangoes make a delicious (if messy) snack when peeled and sliced. Mango slices also can be added to green salad and fruit smoothies or baked in pies.

●**Kiwifruit**—fuzzy brown outside, brilliant green inside—is packed with vitamin C. The kiwifruit is a natural blood thinner that reduces blood levels of *triglycerides* (fats). Peel and slice to eat alone, add to a fruit salad or blend into a smoothie.

●**Apricots** are rich in vitamin A and healthful plant pigments called *carotenoids* (such as beta-carotene and *lycopene*), which aid vision. Lycopene also may fight heart disease and prostate problems.

●**Apples** provide fiber plus heart-healthy *quercetin*. Slice and spread with almond butter (for protein), or sprinkle with cinnamon (to balance blood sugar).

•**Bananas** are rich in potassium, to maintain normal blood pressure and heart function…and provide B vitamins, which help to balance brain chemicals called *neurotransmitters*. Our after-dinner snack often consists of bananas with cinnamon or peanut butter.

•**Blueberries** contain purplish pigments called *anthocyanins* (also found in red grapes and cranberries), which fight urinary tract infections and may protect the brain from oxidative stress, reducing the effects of dementia. Blueberries have vitamin E and other nutrients that strengthen blood vessels.

•**Oranges** have more than 170 phytonutrients and more than 60 *flavonoids* (healthful plant pigments) that fight inflammation, blood clots and various cancers. Other citrus fruits provide similar benefits.

•**Avocados** are rich in *oleic acid*, a monounsaturated fat that lowers LDL "bad" cholesterol. Peel and slice them into salads, add them to burritos, or mash as a sandwich spread.

BODY-BUILDING PROTEINS

Protein is required for muscle and tissue repair, blood sugar balance and proper immune function.

•**Eggs** we buy are organic (laid by chickens that eat grains free of chemicals and that are not treated with hormones or antibiotics) and enriched with omega-3 fatty acids for cardiovascular health. We each have three to five eggs weekly—boiled, poached or scrambled with cheese.

•**Poultry** (skin removed) is typically lower in saturated fat than red meat and therefore is healthier for the cardiovascular system. We select poultry labeled "free range" (meaning the animals were not constrantly caged and were not fed antibiotics). From the deli counter, we buy cooked, sliced turkey and chicken breast for sandwiches, opting for low-sodium, preservative-free brands. Favorite dinner entrées include turkey loaf (ground turkey can be substituted for beef and pork in meat loaf recipes) and pan-fried or broiled turkey burgers. We also love Angela's baked chicken breasts, seasoned with rosemary, lemon and poultry seasoning.

We seldom barbecue meat or poultry because doing so creates cancer-causing compounds called *heterocyclic amines* (HCAs).

•**Wild ocean salmon** (which we consider to be more healthful than farm-raised) we buy when it is in season, to bake or broil with olive oil and lemon. In addition to being low in calories and saturated fat, salmon is high in protein…omega-3s…vitamins B-3, B-6 and B-12 (cobalamin)…phosphorous…and magnesium. We avoid tuna—including canned—due to concerns about mercury contamination. However, canned ocean salmon packed in water is healthful, as are canned sardines—though I confess that we do not enjoy the taste (or smell) of sardines.

•**Cheeses** we enjoy in moderation include Colby and string cheese for snacks and shredded cheddar on burritos. Along with protein and calcium, cheese provides the amino acid *tryptophan*, which promotes thyroid function and positive moods.

CANS, CARTONS & JARS

Packaged goods can be healthful, provided they don't have added preservatives, oils, sugars or salt.

•**Beans** are a must for Mexican-style tostados. Their soluble fiber promotes proper cholesterol and blood sugar levels. Black beans are rich in antioxidant anthocyanins. Pinto beans have magnesium, potassium, manganese, copper and *molybdenum*, which help the liver with detoxification.

•**Almond milk** is rich in potassium. Blue Diamond's unsweetened almond milk tastes great in cereal and scrambled eggs. A sweetened brand called Almond Breeze has 7 grams (g) of sugar per eight-ounce serving. We pour it over hot oatmeal and drink it as a snack. We also buy oat milk and rice milk. (We avoid drinking cow's milk because it can cause allergic and immune reactions and digestive distress.)

•**Peanut butter** is a passion for our kids (and our dog, Blast). We buy pure peanut butter (in a glass container to avoid chemicals that may leach from plastics) that has no added sugar or partially hydrogenated fat. Peanut butter has heart-healthy monounsaturated fats, vitamin E, niacin, folate, manganese and *resveratrol* (the same antioxidant found in red wine). We also like almond butter, which is similar in nutrient content.

GREAT GRAINS & OTHER GOODIES

Selecting grains can be complicated for people who—like my youngest son and me—experience nasal congestion, bloating and diarrhea after consuming foods with *gluten* (a protein complex). Wheat, rye and barley all contain gluten.

•**Gluten-free grains** include corn, amaranth, rice, buckwheat and quinoa. Of the gluten-free breads we have tried, those from Kinnikinnick Foods (877-503-4466, *www.kinnikinnick.com*) taste best. Pastas, cereals, pretzels, corn chips, tortillas and tostado shells also come in gluten-free varieties.

•**Cereals** we select have no more than 3 g of sugar and provide at least 2 g to 3 g of fiber per serving. Favorites include Rice Crunch-Ems from Health Valley…Amazon Frosted Flakes from Nature's Path…and Kix or Cheerios from General Mills. We also get oatmeal—a source of energy-sustaining complex carbohydrates, as well as manganese, *selenium* and *silicon*, which promote bone and cartilage health. The slow-cooking kind has the most fiber.

•**Seeds and nuts** are on our list, too. I grind up two tablespoons of flaxseeds each morning, place them on my tongue, and wash them down with water. Flaxseeds provide fiber and essential fatty acids, and may combat cancer. Hemp seeds are high in protein and omega-3s. Almonds and walnuts are rich in antioxidants and omega-3s, respectively. Angela and I eat one-quarter cup daily, and we try to get our kids to eat a few.

•**Chips** are big hits, especially bruschetta chips from Wild Oats (800-494-9453, *www.wildoats products.com*). Made with potatoes, tomatoes, basil and olive oil, they provide protein and fiber but no sugar or saturated fat.

•**Oils** are important to good cooks (like Angela). Extra-virgin olive oil is what we use when cooking fish and chicken or roasting vegetables. Its monounsaturated fats promote cardiovascular health. To scramble eggs, we use organic canola oil, which contains vitamin E and omega-3s. Macadamia nut oil is best for stir-frying because it has a higher *smoke point* (the temperature at which a cooking oil breaks down and smokes, giving food an unpleasant taste).

•**Fun foods** we enjoy without guilt include Rice Dream Bars (ice cream bars made from rice milk)…Newman's Own brand fig cookies…Ghirardelli semisweet chocolate chips…and SunSpire carob chips.

Eating healthfully comes at a premium. The price of organic foods is about 25% higher than the cost of foods that may have been grown using pesticides or made with unhealthful processing methods. We are happy to pay the price because our family's health is worth it. I suspect you feel the same way.

WHAT WE WON'T BUY

We check labels and stay away from…

•**Artificial sweeteners** (sucralose, aspartame and saccharin), which may cause headaches, rashes and mood changes.

•**High-fructose corn syrup,** which contains many calories but no nutritional benefit.

•**Monosodium glutamate (MSG),** a salty "flavor enhancer" that can cause headaches and/or digestive upset.

•**Partially hydrogenated fats,** also called trans fats, which harm the cardiovascular and immune systems.

•**Sodium nitrate and potassium nitrate,** preservatives that are linked to cancer.

Natural Ways to Fight Prostate Enlargement

If you're a man approaching age 45, you have a nearly 50% chance of having an enlarged prostate. By age 70, the chances are almost nine in 10 that you'll have it. Called *benign prostatic hyperplasia* (BPH), the condition involves an enlarged prostate that compresses the urethra and partially blocks urine flow. BPH is the most common prostate problem among men. While it's not life-threatening—it is not, for example, related to the development of prostate cancer—symptoms can be troublesome. Fortunately, there are natural ways to prevent and treat it.

THE PROSTATE PRESSURE POINT

The job of the prostate is to produce fluid that nourishes and transports sperm. This walnut-sized gland weighs approximately 20 grams, about as much as two Fig Newtons. Located in front of the rectum and below the bladder, the prostate surrounds the urethra, the passageway that carries urine away from the bladder and into the penis.

A swollen prostate can compress the urethra like a clamp on a garden hose, restricting urine flow. It also may press upward, irritating the outer wall of the bladder. This irritation makes the bladder wall thicker and even more easily irritated. A man with BPH might start having bladder contractions, making him feel the need to urinate frequently even when there's not much urine. Over time, the bladder may lose the ability to completely empty, increasing discomfort.

POSSIBLE CAUSES

There remains a lot to be answered when it comes to the causes of BPH. One thing researchers can agree on is that hormonal factors play the largest role.

Research has focused on the hormone *testosterone* and a related substance called *dihydrotestosterone* (DHT). Some researchers believe that testosterone, an anabolic (growth-promoting) hormone, is the main culprit. Others disagree because prostate growth tends to be a problem later in a man's life, while the amount of testosterone is at its highest when males are in their late teens or early 20s.

The conversion of testosterone to DHT increases as men get older—and DHT is very potent. It stimulates the proliferation of new prostate cells and slows the death of older ones. But if DHT is a cause, why do some men with prostate enlargement have normal DHT levels? Could another hormone be involved?

Now researchers are looking at the effect of the hormone *estrogen* (especially the kind called *estradiol*) on prostate growth. Estrogen isn't just a "female" hormone. Men have it as well, and as they age, estrogen levels increase. High estrogen-to-testosterone ratios could increase the effects of DHT on prostate cells.

LOOKING FOR TROUBLE

The most common test to diagnose BPH and other prostate-related problems is a digital rectal exam. Your physician inserts a gloved finger into the rectum and feels the part of the prostate next to the rectum for any enlargement or hardness. All men over age 40 should have this test once a year.

A variety of pharmaceuticals can help relieve BPH symptoms, but each has potential side effects. Many doctors prescribe alpha-blockers, such as *terazosin* (Hytrin) or *doxazosin* (Cardura), which relax the neck of the bladder, making urination easier—but these can cause fatigue, weakness, headaches and dizziness. Another prescription drug, *finasteride* (Proscar), relieves symptoms by shrinking the prostate gland, but it can cause impotence and reduced sexual desire.

For men who have serious BPH problems that are interfering with their lifestyle, some doctors recommend surgical procedures—but surgery can lead to impotence or incontinence.

I find that drugs and surgery usually are unnecessary. As long as a man is getting his prostate checked at least once a year and there are no signs of tumor growth or urinary blockage, BPH can be treated with natural therapies. These include improved diet and supplements. Also, 30 minutes of daily exercise has been shown to reduce BPH symptoms quite significantly.

HEALING FOODS

•**Avocados** contain *beta sitosterol*, a phytonutrient that protects against prostate enlargement by inhibiting growth factors that cause prostate swelling. Avocados also are a good source of *oleic acid*, a monounsaturated fatty acid that is thought to reduce inflammation, which can contribute to BPH. Have at least two weekly servings (one-fifth of a medium avocado per serving). If you don't like avocados, you can have three half-cup servings a week of peanuts, rice bran or wheat germ.

•**Fish** is a good source of *eicosapentaenoic acid* (EPA), a powerful omega-3 fatty acid that helps reduce swelling and inflammation. Eat at least two three-ounce servings of trout, salmon or sardines each week.

•**Ground flaxseed** has been shown to reduce estrogen levels, and it contains anti-inflammatory omega-3 fatty acids. I advise men to take one or two tablespoons daily along with 10 ounces of water (to prevent constipation). As I have noted on several occasions, ground flaxseed has a mild, nutty flavor and can be added to salads, cereals, yogurt, smoothies and protein shakes or just eaten plain.

•**Pumpkin seeds** are natural sources of zinc. This mineral helps keep your prostate healthy by reducing the activity of the enzyme *5-alpha-reductase*, which produces DHT. Sprinkle a tablespoon or two of pumpkin seeds—raw or roasted, with or without the hulls—on salad, yogurt, cereal, etc. four times weekly.

•**Soy** contains a number of phytoestrogens (plant chemicals that balance estrogen), including *genistein*, which can help control prostate enlargement. I prefer fermented soy foods, such as miso, tempeh and fermented soy protein powder, which provide a form of genistein that can be readily absorbed by the body. Have at least one-half cup serving daily.

•**Tomatoes** are rich in the disease-fighting antioxidants known as *carotenoids*. Preliminary scientific research has suggested that tomatoes and tomato products help prevent prostate cancer. They also may have a beneficial effect on prostate enlargement. Consume two servings of fresh tomatoes and two servings of cooked tomatoes (e.g., tomato paste/sauce) weekly (one serving equals one-half to one cup of tomatoes and/or tomato sauce). If you don't like tomatoes, eat watermelon or cantaloupe.

Foods to avoid: Men with BPH should avoid caffeinated beverages and alcohol—they irritate and inflame the prostate. Also reduce your intake of foods that contain harmful fats, such as hydrogenated or partially hydrogenated oils, that promote inflammation. Stay away from packaged foods that are high in sugar, which also can worsen inflammation.

NATURAL SUPPLEMENTS

The following supplements are listed in order of importance—start with the first and move down the list until you find what works best for you. Many formulas contain a blend of two or three of the ones listed.

•**Saw palmetto berry extract** is a mainstay in the natural treatment of BPH and alleviates most symptoms. It was first used medicinally by Native Americans for prostate and urinary tract problems. Recently, researchers have found that saw palmetto helps the prostate by reducing activity of the DHT-producing enzyme 5-alpha-reductase. A review of 18 randomized, controlled trials involving 2,939 men found saw palmetto to be as effective as the BPH drug finasteride.

It can take six to eight weeks before this natural prostate protector begins to fully take effect. I recommend a product that is standardized to contain 80% to 95% fatty acids (check the label) and a total daily dosage of 320 mg, which can be taken all at once. Two brands I recommend are Nature's Way Standardized Saw Palmetto Extract and Enzymatic Therapy Super Saw Palmetto, which are widely available at health-food stores. It is best to take it on an empty stomach. A small percentage of men get stomach upset from saw palmetto. If this occurs, try taking it with meals.

•**Pygeum africanum,** an extract that comes from the bark of the African plum tree, decreases the need to urinate at night and improves urine flow during the day. I prefer a formula that combines pygeum with saw palmetto, such as Ultra Saw Palmetto + Pygeum by Jarrow Formulas (*www.jarrow.com,* or call 800-726-0886 to locate a store near you). The daily pygeum dosage is 100 mg.

•**Nettle root** can provide modest benefits. The nettle-containing product from Nutrilite, Saw Palmetto with Nettle Root, produced good results in a UCLA study. Over six months, the 44 men in the study showed modest improvements in BPH symptoms. The Nutrilite formula includes saw palmetto, nettle root, beta-carotene, pumpkin seed oil and lemon bioflavonoid concentrate (Nutrilite, 800-253-6500, to find a store near you, *www.nutrilite.com*). Take one softgel three times daily.

•**Pollen extracts** seem to relax the muscles of the urethra and improve the ability of the bladder to contract. The extract most widely tested is PollenAid (877-472-6469, *www.nutrilite.com*). Take three capsules daily before meals with a glass of water.

•**Fish oil** can help reduce prostate swelling and inflammation. Take 3,000 mg to 5,000 mg daily in addition to two weekly servings of fish. If you prefer a vegetarian source of omega-3 fatty acids, use one to two tablespoons of flaxseed oil.

Caution: Fish oil should not be used by anyone who takes blood-thinning medications such as *warfarin* (Coumadin).

COMMON SYMPTOMS OF BPH

- **A need to urinate frequently**
- **Urination that is hard to start or stop**
- **Weak urination or "dribbling"**
- **Sensation of an incompletely emptied bladder**
- **Increased need to urinate at night**
- **Burning pain accompanying urination**
- **Recurring bladder infections**

What I Do to Stay Healthy And Live Longer

Terry Grossman, MD, founder and medical director of Frontier Medical Institute, an internationally renowned antiaging and longevity clinic in Denver. www.fmiclinic.com. His books include The Baby Boomers' Guide to Living Forever (Hubristic).

We are on the verge of radically extending human life. Within a few decades, a single drop of blood will detect cancer at its earliest stages or reveal preventable diseases that we might otherwise develop later in life. Medicine will be customized, with drugs and therapies that match our genetic makeup. It will be common to maintain a high quality of life into our 90s and 100s.

Our challenge today is to stay healthy so that we can benefit from this revolution. We all know how important it is to watch our weight, cholesterol and blood pressure, but that's not enough. I counsel patients on optimal management of the aging process—and I practice what I preach. *Here's what I'm doing to increase my chances of living longer...*

TAKE ADVANTAGE OF GENETIC TESTING

For about $500 (not covered by insurance), you can get tests that show your predisposition to such conditions as high blood pressure, heart attack, Alzheimer's disease and osteoporosis.

What I do: I'm in my 60s, and genomic testing revealed that I have a gene that gives me a 250% greater risk of Alzheimer's than the general population. The results depressed me for several days, but they motivated me to fine-tune my health. For example, I take supplements* to nourish my brain. I recommend these supplements to most of my patients, but especially those who are at higher risk for Alzheimer's. Always check with your doctor before taking any supplement.

Brain nutrients I take daily: 20 milligrams (mg) of vinpocetine (pronounced *vinn-POH-seh-teen*), a nutrient derived from the periwinkle plant that increases blood flow to the brain and has memory-enhancing effects...100 mg of phosphatidylserine, a substance that slows memory loss and is found in the cell membranes of body tissue...500 mg twice a day of acetyl-l-carnitine (pronounced *ah-SEE-til-el-CAR-nih-teen*), an amino acid that boosts brain metabolism...100 mg of ginkgo biloba, a tree leaf popular in Chinese medicine that increases cerebral circulation (ginkgo should be avoided by people on blood thinners, such as aspirin or Coumadin).

To find a doctor or facility that performs genetic testing and offers counseling, contact the American College for Advancement in Medicine, 800-532-3688, *www.acam.org.*

GET BODY FAT UNDER 15%

Some fat tissue is necessary. Fat is the body's primary form of energy and is necessary to cushion vital organs. Too much fat, however, secretes inflammatory chemicals that age your body. Reducing body fat is more important than losing weight.

To determine your percentage of body fat, you can purchase a...

- **Body-fat test caliper,** such as the Accu-Measure Fitness 3000 Personal Body Fat Tester, available for $20 at *www.accumeasurefitness.com* or 800-866-2727. This is fairly accurate.

- **Some scales also measure body fat.** They are more accurate than a caliper but also more expensive. See the Body Composition Monitor with scale HBF-500 at *www.omronhealthcare.com* or 800-634-4350.

What I do: At six feet tall and 178 pounds, I score very well on all the height/weight charts,

*Supplements mentioned in this article are available at most health-food stores.

but my body fat percentage is 17.9%. I would like to lose eight more pounds to reach my target of 15% body fat.

I keep my carbohydrate intake under 30% of total calories and emphasize fish, lean meats, vegetables, tofu and miso soup. This is similar to the diet of people in the Okinawa region of Japan, which has more 100-year-olds than any place in the world and very little serious disease.

Helpful book: *The Okinawa Program: How the World's Longest-Lived People Achieve Everlasting Health—and How You Can Too*, written by Bradley J. Willcox, D. Craig Willcox and Makoto Suzuki (Three Rivers).

INCREASE ALKALINITY

Our bodies continually produce toxic waste in the form of acid (lactic acid, uric acid and fatty acids), which needs to be removed from the blood or neutralized.

Example: While many people believe that kidney stones are caused by excess calcium, the real culprit is a high level of phosphoric acid, a primary ingredient in carbonated soft drinks.

What I do: Drink four cups of green tea daily for its alkalinizing effect and antioxidants…and avoid soda.

ELIMINATE SUGAR

Sweets, fructose, corn syrup and high-glycemic-load carbohydrates (pasta, doughnuts, etc.) are the biggest villains in the aging process. Sugar creates a vicious cycle that wears down the body's cells—it spikes the level of insulin in your blood, which causes an intense craving for even more sugar. I don't recommend artificial sweeteners because of the negative long-term effects.

What I do: Use stevia, a noncaloric herb that lowers blood sugar and kills the bacteria that cause tooth decay. It has been used in Paraguay for centuries with no health dangers and can be found in health-food stores as a dietary supplement. (The FDA has not approved its use as a food additive.)

OPTIMIZE TOXIN REMOVAL

Methylation is a simple biochemical process that the body uses to rid itself of dangerous toxins. Between 10% and 44% of the population has a problem with proper methylation, which can lead to cancer, stroke and other conditions.

In a healthy person, methylation neutralizes homocysteine—a toxic by-product that forms after you eat protein. Homocysteine can damage arteries, and high levels are associated with heart attack, Alzheimer's, stroke and cancer.

What I do: I get tested for homocysteine (the test costs $50 to $100). My level is excellent—below 7.5—but if it should rise, I would lower it with daily supplements, including 50 micrograms (mcg) to 100 mcg of vitamin B-6…100 mcg or more of vitamin B-12…and 800 mcg or more of folic acid. These dosages are much higher than the FDA recommendation, so check with your doctor.

REDUCE INFLAMMATION

Whenever its equilibrium is disrupted by injury or infection, the body responds with acute inflammation, such as in muscles and tendons. While this acute inflammation usually subsides quickly, "silent" inflammation can smolder in your body for decades without causing any obvious problems.

Example: Silent inflammation in the coronary arteries is the reason why many seemingly healthy people suddenly drop dead of heart attacks. People with high inflammation readings suffer more than twice the rate of heart attacks as those with low readings.

What I do: Take a blood test (less than $50) for high-sensitivity C-reactive protein (CRP). CRP is made in the liver and released into the blood in response to body inflammation. A normal CRP level is under 3, but for optimal health, it should be under 1. To achieve that, I eat at least four servings of fish per week. Fish and shellfish, such as sole, halibut, catfish, cod, flounder, crab, salmon and shrimp, are rich in omega-3 fatty acids and help reduce inflammation. Other foods that decrease inflammation include walnuts, spinach, broccoli, kale and such spices and herbs as turmeric and rosemary. I also take fish oil capsules (2,100 mg of EPA and 1,500 mg of DHA a day).

INVOKE THE RELAXATION RESPONSE

That's what Harvard Medical School researchers call the meditative state that reduces blood levels of stress hormones, such as cortisol and adrenaline. Long-term exposure to these hormones can lead to osteoporosis, high blood pressure, cataracts and other health problems.

What I do: I attend an hour-long yoga class three times a week. The relaxing stretches help lower my blood pressure and improve my sleep and gastrointestinal functioning.

Gingerroot—Not Just For Cookies

For centuries, ginger (*Zingiber officinale*) has been widely valued as a medicinal herb. It is one of the most widely prescribed herbs by practitioners of Ayurvedic and Chinese traditional medicines. The botanical name for ginger is zingiber, which, in Sanskrit, means "shaped like a horn." Technically speaking, the root is actually a rhizome, a stem that runs underneath the surface of the ground.

It's most commonly used to treat digestive disorders and arthritis in all the healing traditions. It is known as a warming herb, especially suited to people with "cold constitutions," and it's said to enhance circulation. Chinese herbalists use fresh ginger to "warm the lung and stomach."

Ginger is prescribed in Chinese medicine for the common cold, flu, coughs, vomiting, nausea and general digestive upset and bleeding. It also reduces the toxicity of other herbs, so it's essentially an antidote to plants that might have side effects. Also, ginger can help protect an intestinal tract that has been ravaged by tainted or toxic food.

To practitioners of traditional Chinese medicine, every form of gingerroot has certain distinct properties. Fresh ginger has a warming effect on the exterior of the body, while the dried ginger is apt to be recommended for warming the middle of the body.

One of the more intriguing Chinese medicine cures is quick-fried ginger, which is made by frying ginger until the surface is slightly blackened. Practitioners say this is the type that's effective for stopping bleeding and treating conditions that affect the lower abdomen.

Today, ginger is used by herbalists and physicians to treat colds, arthritis, digestive conditions, respiratory-tract infections, headaches, motion sickness and cardiovascular disease.

As with many herbs, ginger has many different active constituents. Dried gingerroot contains between 1% and 4% volatile oils, which account for the strong taste and aroma. (The volatile oils include bisabolene, zingiberene and zingiberol.) Two of the pungent principles—gingerol and shogaol—are believed to be responsible for a lot of the medicinal effects.

Ginger also contains proteolytic enzymes that help to digest proteins and reduce inflammation. Many commercial products are standardized to the constituent gingerol.

DIGESTIVE POWER

Ginger has the unique ability to improve many organs that are involved with digestion. Known as an *aromatic bitter,* it tonifies the intestinal muscles and stimulates the digestive organs. It also stimulates secretion of bile from the liver and gallbladder, which helps digest fats. Ginger is also a well-known carminative, meaning that it can reduce gas and bloating.

ANTI-INFLAMMATORY

Ginger acts as a natural anti-inflammatory by inhibiting the release of prostaglandins and other chemicals in the body that promote inflammation and pain. Unlike nonsteroidal medications such as aspirin, it does not have the potential to damage the stomach, liver and kidneys. For centuries, people used ginger as an anti-inflammatory without knowing how or why it worked. Modern tests have now proven the herb's anti-inflammatory powers.

CIRCULATION AND CARDIOVASCULAR HEALTH

Ginger promotes cardiovascular health by making platelets (cells responsible for blood clots) less likely to clump together. This action allows the blood to keep flowing smoothly and helps prevent hardening of the arteries.

Studies have shown that this protective effect is achieved by inhibiting the formation of thromboxanes, substances that promote blood clotting. Other substances in ginger promote the synthesis of prostacyclin, a component that helps prevent platelets from "aggregating" or clumping together.

Animal studies have also shown that ginger improves the pumping ability of the heart.

Dosage: Fresh gingerroot can be made into tea. It's also sold in capsules, tablets and tinctures. I have found all these forms to work with patients and myself.

The tea is relaxing and works well for digestive upset, as do the capsule and tincture forms. For the treatment of inflammatory conditions, I recommend a standardized capsule to get high levels of the active constituents that reduce inflammation.

The typical capsule dosage is 500 milligrams two to four times daily. If you're taking the tincture, I recommend 20 to 30 drops two to three times daily.

What are the side effects?: Side effects are rare with ginger, though some people (my wife among them!) report heartburn after taking it. In the short term, pregnant women can take ginger for nausea and vomiting related to morning sickness. One to two grams appear to be safe and effective.

Ginger stimulates bile production, so some herbal experts recommend that you should avoid this herb if you have gallstones.

Although I have seen no human studies on drug interactions and ginger, it theoretically may cause a problem with blood-thinning medications such as Coumadin. So check with your physician before using high doses of ginger if you are on a blood-thinning medication.

One last piece of advice you may not find in many books is that gingerroot by itself may aggravate those who are very warm-blooded. If you are the type of person who gets warm and sweats easily, then long-term use of ginger is not recommended just because it can cause discomfort by making you even warmer.

Recommendations for…

•**Arthritis.** Many herbal medicine experts mention that ginger is effective in treating arthritis, but in day-to-day treatment of patients, I have not found this to be true. Ginger by itself does not usually provide substantial relief. That said, however, it can be helpful to some people as part of a comprehensive herbal formula, such as practitioners of Chinese herbal formulas have created for patients with a "cold constitution."

•**Bloating and flatulence.** Ginger is the remedy par excellence for relieving bloating and flatulence, which is the common result of what I call SAD (Standard American Diet). It reminds me of one lady who came up to me after a talk, looked around to make sure no one else was listening, and asked if there was anything I could recommend for her 36-year-old son who was having trouble with a lot of gas. It turns out this son was newly married, and his mother was worried that his flatulence would cause marital problems.

I recommended she give her son a bottle of ginger capsules to use with meals. Hopefully it rescued the young groom from some embarrassment—or possibly saved the marriage!

•**Cardiovascular disease.** Since ginger is a natural blood thinner, it promotes good circulation and therefore improves cardiovascular health. Animal studies show that it helps with the pumping action of the heart. To me, it is most beneficial as a synergistic herb—one that makes other herbs more effective rather than working by itself.

•**Diarrhea.** There's a specific type of diarrhea, called *cold diarrhea* in Chinese medicine, that ginger seems to help significantly. This is the kind that gives you a case of the chills as well as loose stools. (What's called *hot diarrhea,* as you might expect, is the kind where loose stools are accompanied by a feeling of feverishness.)

•**High cholesterol.** In animal studies, ginger has been found to lower cholesterol levels in rats. Unfortunately, it doesn't show exactly the same effect in humans. But if you're taking ginger for other conditions, there is a possibility that it could also help lower your cholesterol.

•**Morning sickness.** Ginger has actually been studied as a relief for severe morning sickness. In 19 of the 27 women who took ginger for nausea and vomiting, both symptoms became less frequent within four days of treatment. The dosage of gingerroot capsules was 250 milligrams taken 4 times daily.

Since publication of the earliest studies, which were done in 1990, many conventional doctors have started to recommend gingerroot for morning sickness. (My wife's obstetrician, for instance, recommends it to her patients.) However, I don't advise that women take more than one gram daily during pregnancy, and there's no reason to continue taking it after the morning sickness passes.

•Motion sickness. Ginger has received a lot of attention for its ability to prevent and treat motion sickness. A study in 1982 revealed that ginger was superior to the drug Dramamine for reducing motion sickness. Not every study, since then, has supported this finding, but some excellent research done in 1994—involving 1,741 people—confirmed that ginger was indeed very effective in treating motion sickness.

The 1994 study was done with a group of people who were taking a whale-watching trip. Before boarding the boat, people were asked to take various kinds of motion-sickness remedies, ginger among them. (None of the passengers knew which remedy they were being given.) The study showed that 250 milligrams of ginger was just as powerful as the pharmaceutical medications, but without side effects such as drowsiness.

•Nausea and vomiting. Bad food, flu, chemotherapy and surgical treatments are just a few of the possible causes of nausea and vomiting. No matter what the cause, however, ginger has been shown to be an effective remedy.

In two studies, ginger helped reduce nausea and vomiting in patients who had just undergone surgery where they received anesthesia. (Anesthesia makes some people very nauseated.) If you are scheduled to have surgery, talk with your surgeon about taking one gram of ginger before and after surgery.

Ultimate Cancer-Fighting Food...Now in Capsule Form, Too

I do not like broccoli. I haven't liked it since I was a little kid and my mother made me eat it. I'm president of the United States, and I'm not going to eat any more broccoli!" George H.W. Bush spoke these words early in his tenure at the White House. Unfortunately, he is missing out on a potent cancer-fighting food.

If you share the former president's aversion to broccoli, you'll be happy to learn of convenient new alternatives that offer even more health benefits. *First, some background information...*

DEFICIENT DIETS

Researchers have published eye-opening studies on the compound *sulforaphane*, found in broccoli and similar vegetables. Sulforaphane helps prevent cancers of the breast, ovary, prostate, bone, brain, bladder, liver, lung and stomach and combats other conditions associated with aging and cell death.

It is no secret that the average American fails to consume the seven to nine daily servings of fruits and vegetables recommended to provide dietary protection against cancer and other diseases. And for many people, the produce they do eat seldom includes the recommended one to two daily servings of *cruciferous* vegetables (so called because the plants' flowers have four petals arranged like a crucifix), such as cauliflower, kale, bok choy, rutabagas, radishes, turnips, brussels sprouts and, of course, broccoli. An analysis published in the *Journal of Nutrition*, which looked at dietary data on 4,806 men and women ages 25 to 75, revealed that just 3% of the group consumed broccoli during either of two typical days. Consumption of dark green vegetables averaged just one-fifth of a serving per day.

Cruciferous vegetables are a rich source of healthful plant chemicals called *phytochemicals* or *phytonutrients*. These include cancer-fighting *thiols* (such as the sulfur-containing *glucosinolates*) and *indoles* (which bind chemical carcinogens and activate detoxifying enzymes). Yet even veggie lovers may find it difficult to ingest therapeutic amounts of cruciferous vegetables on a regular basis. This problem is compounded by the fact that cooking can destroy phytonutrients, so health benefits are diminished unless the vegetables are consumed raw or lightly steamed.

SGS DISCOVERED

Scientists at Johns Hopkins University School of Medicine identified the compound *sulforaphane glucosinolate* (SGS)—a naturally occurring precursor to sulforaphane—in 1992 and began to research its cancer-fighting potential. Leading this effort was Paul Talalay, MD, a professor of pharmacology and director of the university's Laboratory for Molecular Sciences.

His strategy: To support the body's natural detoxification capacity to fight cancer-causing chemicals and cell-damaging free radicals. It is well accepted that cell DNA controls replication of cells and that damage to cell DNA is an important factor in the development of cancer.

In 1994, Dr. Talalay looked at the impact of SGS on mammary (breast) tumors in rats exposed to a potent carcinogen. Results were astounding. The number of rats that developed tumors was reduced by as much as 60%...the number of tumors in each animal was reduced by 80%...and the size of the tumors that did develop was reduced by 75%. Subsequently, hundreds of other test tube and animal studies have confirmed the anticancer properties of sulforaphane.

Toxins (natural and man-made) go through phases of breakdown in the cells of the body, particularly the liver. *Sulforaphane promotes detoxification by...*

•**Supporting enzymes that destroy carcinogens.**

•**Stimulating longer-lasting protective antioxidant effects** than other nutrients do.

•**Replenishing the cells' levels of the amino acid *glutathione,*** strengthening the immune system.

•**Inhibiting COX-2,** an inflammatory enzyme that contributes to cancerous changes in cells.

•**Limiting DNA damage and abnormal cell growth.**

SUPER SPROUTS

Dr. Talalay discovered that various types of fresh and frozen broccoli differed significantly in the amounts of SGS they contained—and that the older the broccoli was, the lower its SGS. Painstaking research uncovered certain varieties of three-day-old broccoli sprouts—which look like a cross between alfalfa sprouts and bean sprouts—that contained up to 50 times more SGS than mature, cooked broccoli. One ounce of these sprouts could provide as much SGS as *three pounds* of cooked broccoli.

This set the stage for a fascinating study, published in *Cancer Epidemiology Biomarkers & Prevention.* The study was conducted in a rural area near Shanghai where liver cancer is common because local grain is contaminated with *aflatoxin,* a carcinogen produced by mold.

In the study, broccoli sprouts with known levels of SGS were grown at the site in China. Three days after the shoots emerged from the soil, the sprouts were picked and used to prepare a liquid extract to ensure standard dosages. One hundred local residents drank five ounces of diluted extract in tea form (equal to eating two ounces of sprouts) daily for two weeks. A control group drank a tea indistinguishable in taste and appearance but containing no SGS.

Great results: Analysis of the participants' urine showed that in people who drank the SGS extract, carcinogens were being removed from the body—providing the first direct evidence that broccoli sprouts can enhance the human body's detoxifying system, reducing the risk of cancer.

NEW WAYS TO GET GREENS

Broccoli sprouts and SGS are safe for everyone. (If you have thyroid problems, check with your doctor—there is a slight risk that broccoli sprouts may suppress thyroid function. There is no concern with the SGS supplement.) Because the SGS content of broccoli sprouts can vary greatly depending on seed type and growing methods, I recommend the sprouts developed by the Johns Hopkins team. These are now available under the brand name BroccoSprouts, from Brassica Protection Products (877-747-1277, *www.broccosprouts.com*). Sold in health-food and grocery stores nationwide, these broccoli sprouts contain standardized and therapeutic amounts of sulforaphane.

Alternatively, you can grow your own sprouts using BroccoSprout seeds. Order from Caudill Seed Company (800-695-2241).

For optimal health, eat one-half cup (one ounce) of BroccoSprouts every other day. Each serving contains 73 mg of SGS. They are most beneficial when eaten raw, so sprinkle them on salads and sandwiches. The taste is similar to that of a radish, with a spicy flavor that results from the release of sulforaphane as you chew. Even people who hate broccoli usually enjoy the tangy taste of broccoli sprouts.

CANCER-PREVENTION PILL

Some people don't have the time—or taste buds—for a full day's worth of fruits and vegetables. That's when the capsule form of the cancer-fighting compound *sulphoraphane glucosinolate* (SGS) comes in handy. I recommend it for people with a family history of cancer…as a complement to ongoing cancer treatments (with your doctor's approval)…for those who have been exposed to toxins…and for all who want to reduce their risk of cancer.

The supplement company Xymogen (*www.xymogen.com*) markets Oncoplex SGS, which contains 30 mg of SGS per capsule. Though it does not require a prescription, it is not sold in health-food stores and usually is purchased through holistic doctors.

In general, I advise taking one capsule daily. If you have had cancer or are undergoing cancer treatment, increase to two to four capsules daily, under the supervision of your doctor.

When Gas Won't Quit

Despite careful dietary practices (you avoid carbonated drinks, coffee and beans and you regularly supplement with Beano and Gas-X) you might continue to find that gassiness can't be avoided.

The problem may lie with your medication. Ask your doctor if any of the drugs you take commonly cause flatulence or digestive upset. Gas may result when digestive bacteria fail to break down foods sufficiently. To fix this, stimulate stomach acid secretion with the herb gentian root. Take 10 to 20 drops of liquid extract (in one ounce of water) or 300 mg in capsule form about 10 minutes before meals. (Do not use gentian if you have an active ulcer.) Also take an equal dose of gingerroot, which acts as a *carminative* (gas reducer) and improves stomach function. For improved digestion, restore friendly bacteria to your digestive tract by eating sauerkraut, kefir and/or yogurt, or by taking a probiotic supplement that contains at least 5 billion colony-forming units (CFU) of *lactobacillus acidophilus* and/or *bifidobacterium*. If gassiness persists after three weeks, consult a holistic doctor for food-intolerance testing—you may have a sensitivity to dairy, grains or other foods.

Poor Circulation

If poor circulation in the legs is of concern to you, consider supplementing with ginkgo biloba. This herb dilates arteries in the limbs.

Dosage: 120 mg of a ginkgo extract (with 24% flavone glycosides and 6% terpene lactones) twice daily for eight weeks. Also take nattokinase, an enzyme extracted from *natto* (a by-product of fermented boiled soybeans), which is a natural blood thinner.

Dosage: 2,000 fibrin units (FU) per day on an empty stomach for eight weeks. Both are sold at health-food stores and generally are safe, but they should not be taken if you use blood-thinning medication, such as aspirin or *warfarin* (Coumadin).

In addition, each day sprinkle one-half teaspoon of cinnamon onto toast or apple slices, or add it to a smoothie. Cinnamon improves circulation by dilating the arteries, can be used indefinitely, is safe for everyone—and is tasty, too.

Pomegranate Juice and Your Heart

The pomegranate recently has been acclaimed for its health benefits. Pomegranate juice, which is available at health-food stores and most grocery stores, contains a blend of powerful, disease-fighting antioxidants, including phenolic compounds, tannins and anthocyanins.

Researchers in Norway found that pomegranates contain a higher concentration of antioxidants than 23 other fruits. This big red fruit has about 10 times more antioxidants than those with the next-highest levels, including grapes, oranges, plums, pineapples, lemons, dates, clementines and grapefruits.

CLEANS YOUR ARTERIES

One of the major benefits of pomegranate juice is that it prevents the oxidation of "bad" low-density lipoprotein (LDL) cholesterol—a major cause of artery damage and subsequent plaque buildup.

For several years, Israeli researchers have studied the protective antioxidant and cardiovascular effects of pomegranate juice. In one of their most recent studies, pomegranate juice was found to reduce oxidation of LDL cholesterol by 40%. In another study, they found that pomegranate juice reduced the buildup of plaque in the carotid (neck) arteries, which supply blood to the brain.

PROTECTS DIABETICS' ARTERIES

Researchers from Shaheed Beheshti University of Medical Sciences in Tehran, Iran, found pomegranate juice to be helpful for people with diabetes. In this study, participants who consumed 40 g (about 1.4 ounces) daily of concentrated pomegranate juice for eight weeks, saw significant reductions in their total cholesterol and LDL cholesterol levels. This definitely is good news for diabetics because elevated blood glucose and insulin levels raise the risk of atherosclerosis.

I recommend that those with carotid stenosis (narrowing of the carotid arteries) and/or diabetes drink at least two ounces and up to eight ounces of 100% pomegranate juice daily. (Those with diabetes should drink no more than two ounces at a time, and take it with meals to slow down blood sugar absorption.)

For people trying to lower their blood pressure and those with a strong family history of heart disease, I recommend eight ounces a day.

You can, of course, dilute it by half with water (as I do) or combine it with other juices, such as grape or cranberry, for better flavor. One widely available brand that I use regularly is R.W. Knudsen Just Pomegranate.

New to the market are pomegranate supplements, which may prove to be a good alternative for people who wish to avoid the calories in pomegranate juice.

Chasteberry for Women

If you were to examine some of the many "women's hormone-balancing" products in health-food stores and pharmacies, you would most likely see chasteberry (also known as *Vitex agnus castus*) listed as an ingredient. It has been recommended for female conditions, including hormone-related acne, fibrocystic breast syndrome, endometriosis, infertility, lactation difficulties, menopausal hot flashes, menstrual disorders, ovarian cysts and uterine fibroids. In other words, it is touted as helping almost all major female conditions.

The herb comes from the berries of the chasteberry tree, actually a shrub found in subtropical climates. The ancient Greeks used chasteberry as a symbol of chastity in young women, hence the name *chasteberry* or *chaste tree*.

HOW IT WORKS

Chasteberry does not contain hormones. It acts on the pituitary gland in the brain to increase the production of *luteinizing hormone* (LH). LH stimulates the ovaries to release eggs, as occurs with ovulation. Ovulation triggers a surge in levels of the hormone *progesterone*. This release of progesterone is important in maintaining a balance with the other major female hormone, *estrogen*. Research has shown that some premenopausal women do not ovulate regularly. This sets the stage for what is known as *estrogen dominance*—too much estrogen relative to progesterone. By helping to normalize progesterone levels, chasteberry promotes hormone balance. This is why it is effective for so many female conditions, including premenstrual syndrome and fibrocystic breast disease as well as uterine fibroids in women of all ages, which are in large part caused by estrogen dominance.

Chasteberry also has been shown to lower levels of the hormone *prolactin*. When elevated, this hormone, which is secreted by the pituitary gland, is associated with premenstrual syndrome, irregular menstrual cycles and infertility.

DOSAGE

For all of these conditions, I commonly recommend 160 mg to 240 mg daily of a 0.6% *aucubin* or 0.5% *agnuside* extract (important active ingredients) in capsule form—available from Enzymatic Therapy (800-783-2286, *www.enzy.com*) and Nature's Answers (sold by Vitacost, 800-381-0759, *www.vitacost.com*). Or I suggest 40 drops of the tincture in four ounces of water, taken once daily.

For best results, chasteberry should be used until the problem is alleviated and then for an additional three months. Women may notice improvements within two menstrual cycles.

Chasteberry often needs to be taken for four to six months or longer for long-standing cases of hormone imbalance that have resulted in infertility, amenorrhea (no menstrual cycles), irregular menstrual cycles or endometriosis.

Mild digestive upset, nausea, headaches and skin rash are infrequent side effects of chasteberry. Stop taking it if they occur.

Chasteberry should not be used by women taking birth control pills or injections. It also should be avoided by those taking drugs that block dopamine receptors, such as the antipsychotic medication *haloperidol* (Haldol).

As with most herbs, chasteberry should be avoided during pregnancy, although it is helpful for lactation in nursing mothers.

Lastly, some women experience an "adjustment phase" during the first few months of taking chasteberry. It is not uncommon for the menstrual cycle to shorten or lengthen, and flow can become lighter or heavier than what it was previously. This adjustment phase almost always normalizes after two to three months of use.

SPECIAL REPORT #2:

Natural Cures That Work Better Than Drugs

Natural Cures That Work Better Than Drugs

Hormones May Be Your Allies in the Weight Wars

Are you fighting a weight-loss battle? By eating a healthful diet and exercising regularly, you can shed some weight—but then it's common to "get stuck." No matter how you modify your diet and exercise regimen, the pounds just stop coming off. What's going on?

Your hormones may be the key. They influence appetite (when and to what degree you desire food)...metabolism (how you convert food to energy)...and insulin sensitivity (the degree to which your cells respond to insulin, which allows your body to use glucose).

If you have hit a plateau—or even have had a reversal—in your weight-loss efforts, it may be time for you to look more closely at your hormone levels.

To start, have them tested by a physician. Hormone levels can be detected from samples of blood, saliva and urine. A knowledgeable holistic doctor will help you interpret the results and choose supplements or other natural solutions that will allow you to lose those additional pounds.

Important factors to consider...

HOW ACTIVE IS YOUR THYROID?

Your body depends on thyroid hormones to regulate your metabolism. These hormones are produced in the butterfly-shaped gland just below your voice box. If thyroid hormones are in short supply, you can expect to gain weight. Assuming that your physician has ruled out any serious thyroid disease that must be treated in its own right, you can start to beat your weight problem by optimizing your thyroid function.

Mark A. Stengler, ND, naturopathic physician in private practice, La Jolla, California...adjunct associate clinical professor at the National College of Natural Medicine, Portland, Oregon...author of many books, including *The Natural Physician's Healing Therapies* and coauthor of *Prescription for Natural Cures* (both from Bottom Line Books)...and author of the *Bottom Line/Natural Healing* newsletter.

Natural solutions: For mild deficiencies—perhaps your levels are just a little off or are normal but you still have classic low thyroid symptoms, such as weight gain, fatigue, cold hands and feet, poor memory—look into one of these daily supplements or, even better, a formula that combines several of them. Take them until symptoms are better, and then taper off. If symptoms return, start taking them again—or have a doctor monitor you. If there is no improvement within four weeks, stop taking the supplements.

•**Bladderwrack** (a type of algae) contains iodine, which the thyroid requires for optimal functioning.

Typical dose: Two or three 500-mg capsules, in divided doses, for a total of 1,000 to 1,500 mg per day.

•**L-tyrosine** (an amino acid) helps the thyroid to manufacture hormones.

Typical dose: 500 mg twice daily on an empty stomach.

•**Homeopathic thyroid** (a minute dose of thyroid hormone or animal thyroid gland) stimulates your thyroid gland to produce hormones. Follow label directions.

•**Thyroid glandular** (an extract derived from animal thyroid tissue, typically that of a sheep) contains amino acids, vitamins and minerals that stimulate hormone production.

Typical dose: One to two capsules or tablets twice daily on an empty stomach.

Best formulas: I recommend Thyroid Support Liquid Phyto-Caps containing Bladderwrack and L-tyrosine from Gaia Herbs (888-831-7780, *www.gaiaherbs.com*) or Solaray's Thyroid Caps, which has L-tyrosine, iodine and thyroid glandular (800-669-8877, *www.nutraceutical.com*).

If your lab tests reveal a severe deficiency, you will be prescribed a thyroid hormone replacement program. Ask your doctor about natural thyroid replacement treatments, such as Armour Thyroid, Westhroid, Nature-Throid and compounded thyroid tablets.

THE POWER OF DHEA

Dehydroepiandrosterone (DHEA) is an adrenal hormone that enhances metabolism. DHEA levels naturally decline with age. A study of 56 men and women at Washington University

School of Medicine found that those who took 50 mg of DHEA daily for six months experienced a reduction in belly fat and visceral fat—the fat that builds up around internal organs—both of which are associated with heart disease, diabetes and other serious illnesses. Insulin levels also dropped significantly, indicating better blood sugar control and insulin sensitivity.

Natural solutions: If testing indicates that your DHEA level is low—less than 100 micrograms (mcg)/dL—take DHEA. If not, take one of the other supplements described below. Have your levels checked every six months.

•**DHEA supplements** increase DHEA levels.

Typical dose: Up to 50 mg once a day. DHEA is available over the counter, but its use should be monitored by a physician. Potential side effects include facial hair growth in women and prostate enlargement in men.

•**Sterols and sterolins** are plant fats that are chemically similar to animal fats but have different biological functions. Sterols and sterolins support DHEA production by the adrenal glands. Moducare Capsules (877-297-7332, *www.modu care.com*) contain both nutrients.

Typical dose: Two capsules in the morning and one before bedtime on an empty stomach.

•**Cordyceps sinensis** (a medicinal mushroom) also helps support DHEA production.

Typical dose: 2,400 mg of a standardized water/ethanol extract of Cordyceps sinensis strain Cs-4.

THE CORTISOL FACTOR

Prolonged elevation of the stress hormone cortisol can contribute to weight gain. High cortisol levels can interfere with normal thyroid function and decrease insulin sensitivity, both of which lead to weight gain.

Natural solutions: Stress-reduction techniques curb your production of stress hormones. My favorite stress relievers include regular exercise, positive mental imagery and prayer.

Your doctor can order a saliva test to measure your cortisol level. *If yours is elevated, consider…*

•**Ashwagandha** (an herb) reduces cortisol levels when taken daily. Look for products containing the patented ingredient Sensoril, which provides optimal concentrations of ashwagandha. Widely available brands include Liquid Anti-Stress Plus Adrenal Support from Life Solutions Natural Products (a company in which I have a financial interest, 800-914-8771, *www.lifesolutionsnp. com*) and Tribulus Complex with Ashwagandha from Jarrow Formulas (800-726-0886, *www.jar row.com*).

If cortisol levels have not come down after two months of taking ashwagandha, try…

•**DHEA,** described above, which also can reduce cortisol levels.

Typical dose: Up to 50 mg daily, taken under a doctor's supervision.

ESTROGEN DOMINANCE

Most women understand the importance of estrogen, but they might not realize that excessive amounts of this hormone can increase body fat and promote fluid retention. Estrogen in women needs to be "balanced out" with progesterone, which has a diuretic (water-excreting) effect. Premenopause, menopause and any health condition that interferes with ovulation (such as polycystic ovarian syndrome) will reduce levels of progesterone and give fat-building estrogen the upper hand. This is one reason why some women gain weight for no apparent reason.

Natural solutions: The nutrient indole 3-carbinol helps the liver metabolize estrogen. It is found in cruciferous vegetables—broccoli, cauliflower, cabbage and kale. I recommend eating at least one plentiful helping of any of these foods each day.

If a saliva, blood or urine test shows that your estrogen level is elevated even after you adopt an indole 3-carbinol–rich diet or if you just don't like to eat the above foods, try these daily supplements…

•**Indole 3-carbinol** helps the body metabolize estrogen.

Typical dose: 300 mg to 400 mg a day.

•**Vitex** (also called chasteberry, derived from the berries grown on the *Vitex agnus castus* tree) has been shown to improve the regularity of ovulation and raise progesterone levels.

Typical dose: 120 mg of a product standardized to 0.6% aucubine or 0.5% agnuside twice daily…or 800 mg of a nonstandardized supplement. Vitex is available from Nature's Way (to find a retailer, call 800-962-8873 or go to *www. naturesway.com*) and Phytopharmica (800-376-7889, *www.phytopharmica.com*).

•**Natural progesterone cream** should be used as directed by your doctor for extreme progesterone deficiencies.

Typical dose: One-quarter teaspoon (20 mg) applied to the skin one or two times daily for two weeks before menstruation (stop when menses begin) or, if menopausal or postmenopausal, applied once daily. Consider Emerita ProGest (to find a retailer, call 800-648-8211 or go to *www.emerita.com*), a good brand that is commonly available in health-food stores.

THE TESTOSTERONE FACTOR

Testosterone, a powerful hormone found in women and men, affects the body's ability to maintain lean muscle mass. It is mainly produced by the ovaries in women and the testes in men. A low level makes it more difficult to tone muscles and lose weight.

Natural solutions…

•**DHEA** is converted by women's bodies into testosterone. If a woman has low DHEA and low testosterone levels, then doctor-supervised supplementation of DHEA, as described previously, may improve both levels.

•**Panax ginseng** may help boost slightly low levels of testosterone in men and women.

Typical dose: 200 mg daily of a product standardized to 5% ginsenosides.

•**Tribulus terrestris** is a plant whose extract may increase testosterone levels in men and women. So far, research has been done mainly with animals, but this herb appears to be safe. Tribulus by Source Naturals (for a retailer, call 800-815-2333 or go to *www.sourcenaturals. com*) is a good choice, as is Life Solutions Natural Products' Liquid Natural Libido Enhancer (800-914-8771, *www.lifesolutionsnp.com*), which contains ginseng and, for a calming effect, passionflower.

•**Natural testosterone** is available by prescription only and should be used when there is a moderate to severe deficiency. I prefer the transdermal gel or cream form, which is applied to the skin, because it requires less metabolism by the liver than pills.

IS INSULIN ON YOUR TEAM?

Blood sugar (glucose) is terrific fuel for an active person, but you need the right level of insulin to transport the sugar from your bloodstream into tissue. A condition known as insulin resistance occurs when cells become less accepting of glucose and insulin levels spike. It is one factor that sets the stage for weight gain.

Natural solutions…

•**High-fiber diet** that includes seven to nine daily servings of fresh vegetables as well as three servings of whole-grain breads and cereals. Nuts, seeds and raw vegetables are especially good to help balance insulin levels. Stay away from simple-sugar food products, such as white breads, pasta, soft drinks, cookies and other sweets. For protein, avoid fatty red meats and favor quality sources, such as legumes, nuts, eggs, fish and poultry.

•**Help yourself to cinnamon!** Research shows that it helps balance blood sugar levels.

•**Eat smaller servings** throughout the day rather than three big meals, so your body metabolizes food more effectively.

•**High-potency multivitamin/mineral supplement.** Everyone should take one daily for general health—it provides nutrients that, among other things, balance insulin levels.

If tests for fasting blood glucose and insulin indicate that you have insulin resistance, try taking all three of these additional supplements daily…

•**Chromium** (a mineral) is particularly important to balance blood sugar levels.

Typical dose: 400 mcg.

•**Alpha lipoic acid** (an enzyme that acts as a powerful antioxidant) reduces levels of insulin and blood sugar.

Typical dose: Up to 200 mg.

•**Fish oil** (an essential fatty acid supplement) improves insulin sensitivity.

Typical dose: One teaspoon daily or a one-gram capsule, three times a day. Nordic Naturals fish oil supplements are widely available and free of mercury and other toxins (to locate a retailer, call 800-662-2544 or go to *www.nordicnaturals.com*).

Caution: If you are taking a blood-thinning medication, such as *warfarin* (Coumadin), check with your doctor before taking fish oil.

ROOT CAUSES OF WEIGHT GAIN

•Poor diet
•Lack of exercise
•Genetic predisposition
•Hormone imbalance
•Neurotransmitter imbalance, such as serotonin deficiency
•Side effects of drugs
•Toxins, such as chemicals (pesticides)
•Psychological reasons, such as stress, anxiety and depression

Chinese Club Moss for Better Memory

Every so often, we learn that an ancient medicinal herb has new and astonishing health benefits. So it is with Chinese club moss. Perhaps you have heard of it by another name—*huperzia* or *Qian ceng ta*—but most people haven't heard of it at all. Yet as the baby boomer population ages, people will be talking a lot about Chinese club moss and its active ingredient, *huperzine A* (HupA).

New finding: HupA improves memory and slows age-related cognitive decline—even in early-stage Alzheimer's disease patients. (Neither HupA nor drugs help much in later stages of Alzheimer's.)

Chinese medicine practitioners have used club moss for centuries as a diuretic and an anti-inflammatory. Two decades ago, a Chinese scientist discovered that an *alkaloid* (an organic compound) in HupA could improve brain function. This sparked many studies, some ongoing, including a clinical trial at the National Institutes of Health.

HupA's cognitive benefits are due mainly to its effects on acetylcholine, a neurotransmitter critical for normal thinking, memory and attention. These mental processes falter when *acetylcholine* production drops or an enzyme called *acetylcholinesterase* (which normally breaks down unused acetylcholine) is overactive, degrading the much needed acetylcholine.

HupA appears to inhibit activity of acetylcholinesterase, thereby sparing acetylcholine. This also is how pharmaceuticals for Alzheimer's work—but several human clinical trials suggest that HupA may be even more effective than the drugs *donepezil* (Aricept) and *tacrine* (Cognex). Animal studies demonstrate that HupA further supports cognitive function by protecting brain cells from damage caused by free radicals (harmful negatively charged molecules), toxins and/or lack of oxygen (for instance, from poor circulation or stroke)…and by reducing formation of *beta-amyloid*, a protein that forms lesions in the brain tissue of Alzheimer's patients.

I began prescribing HupA eight years ago for patients with memory problems—and many have been delighted with their improvement. HupA seems to work better than *ginkgo biloba*, an herb that increases blood flow to the brain. For ability to improve brain function, on a scale of one to 10, I rate ginkgo at six and HupA at nine. And unlike ginkgo, HupA is safe for people who take blood thinners, such as aspirin or *warfarin* (Coumadin).

For intermittent problems with short-term memory, I recommend that adults under age 55 take 50 micrograms (mcg) to 100 mcg of HupA daily…and that those age 55 and older take 100 mcg twice daily. For more severe memory problems, such as in early Alzheimer's, take 200 mcg twice daily.

HupA is generally safe and can be taken indefinitely. Occasional side effects include nausea, diarrhea, dizziness and/or loss of appetite. Before starting HupA, talk to your doctor. Do not take HupA if you have a cardiac condition that affects heart rate, such as *bradycardia* (slow resting heart rate) or congestive heart failure, because HupA can decrease heart rate and lead to fainting. If you take medication for Alzheimer's disease, do not use HupA, because it might worsen the drug's side effects (nausea, vomiting and sweating). If you are dissatisfied with the Alzheimer's drugs you are taking, ask your doctor about discontinuing them and trying HupA instead.

Huperzine A brands I like include Source Naturals (800-815-2333, *www.sourcenaturals.com*), sold at health-food stores and on-line (for instance, at *www.iherb.com*)…and Ceriva by Metagenics (800-692-9400, *www.metagenics.com*), available from health-care practitioners. Cost runs about $10 per month at a dose of 100 mcg daily. In my view, that's a small price to pay for improved memory and clearer thinking.

Breakthrough Treatments For Hair Loss

Why do some men go bald in their 30s while others have a full head of hair until their final days? Why do some women have ever-thinning hair, while others never seem to lose a single strand?

Blame your genes, first of all. If your mom, dad or a grandparent had hair loss, chances are greater that you will, too. Even so, there are ways to slow hair loss and stimulate growth.

THE HORMONE FACTOR

You grow and shed hair all the time. Of the 100,000-plus strands of hair on your head, it is perfectly normal to lose 50 to 100 every day. Once a hair is shed, a new hair grows from the same follicle. Hair grows at a rate of nearly one-half inch per month (faster in warm weather, slower when frost is on the vine). Baldness results when the rate of shedding exceeds the rate of regrowth.

Hair loss usually accelerates when you're over age 50. One hormone, *dihydrotestosterone* (DHT), seems to be the chief culprit. DHT is a derivative of testosterone (the sex-determining hormone that is more abundant in men than women). In both men and women, DHT increases in the presence of the enzyme *5-alpha reductase*, which is produced in the prostate, adrenal glands and the scalp. 5-alpha reductase is more likely to proliferate after age 50. When DHT is overproduced, hair follicles are damaged. Some follicles die, but most shrink and produce thinner, weaker hairs—and the weak hairs are the ones that fall out.

An oily skin substance called *sebum*—produced by the sebaceous glands—makes matters worse. Excess sebum clogs follicles and contributes to high 5-alpha reductase activity, which stimulates production of DHT.

STRESS

Among my own patients, stress is a factor for both men and women. I have found that highly stressed women, in particular, have higher-than-normal levels of *cortisol*, a stress hormone that can contribute to hair loss.

A study published in the *Journal of Clinical Biochemistry* confirms that cortisol is indeed elevated in some women who suffer hair loss—and that when they learn to cope better with stress, hair growth improves.

For stress relief, I recommend daily exercise, such as brisk walking, as well as relaxation techniques, including deep breathing and meditation. B vitamins and *ashwagandha* (a stress-reducing herb from India) also can help counteract the effects of cortisol.

A regular daily dose of 100 mg of a B-vitamin complex and 250 mg to 500 mg of ashwagandha can help control cortisol levels. Look for Sensoril Ashwagandha, a patented extract formula by Jarrow Formulas, available at many health-food stores or by calling 800-726-0886 or at *www.jarrow.com.*

A PROMISING FORMULA

Taking a daily multivitamin and mineral supplement as well as the herbal remedy saw palmetto also can help slow hair loss. A daily scalp massage with essential oils is beneficial, too.

•**Saw palmetto** helps block the effects of DHT on hair follicles, strengthening hair. In a study in the *Journal of Alternative and Complementary Medicine*, researchers used a product containing saw palmetto and a plant compound called *beta-sitosterol* that is found in saw palmetto and other plants. The study included 19 men between ages 23 and 64 who had mild-to-moderate hair loss. Men in one group were given a placebo daily...and men in the other group received the saw palmetto/beta-sitosterol combination (none of the participants knew which group they were in). After five months, researchers found that 60% of the men who received the saw palmetto/beta-sitosterol combination showed improvement, while only 11% of the men receiving a placebo had more hair growth.

In my clinical experience, saw palmetto is helpful for both men and women. I recommend 320 mg to 400 mg daily of an 85% liposterolic

extract. It is safe to use long term but should not be taken if you are pregnant or nursing.

For a more aggressive approach, you should also take beta-sitosterol. Source Naturals (800-815-2333, *www.sourcenaturals.com*) offers a 113-mg tablet that can be taken daily. It is available at health-food stores and at *www.iherb.com.*

•**The essential oils of rosemary and lavender** have been shown to improve hair growth when applied to the scalp. My own belief is that they improve blood flow to the scalp, ensuring that nutrients get to the sites where they're needed.

You can purchase these essential oils in separate containers. Pour some of your regular shampoo into the lid of the shampoo bottle, then add five to 10 drops of each essential oil. Massage into the scalp and leave on three to five minutes before rinsing thoroughly.

OTHER SUPPLEMENTS

If you have tried these approaches for two to three months and still aren't satisfied with the growth of your locks, here are some other supplements that can help both men and women...

•**Biotin,** a nutrient that is required for hair growth, is particularly good for brittle hair. Food sources of biotin include brewer's yeast, soybeans, eggs, mushrooms and whole wheat. For supplementation, take 3,000 micrograms daily for at least two months or use a biotin-enriched shampoo daily.

•**MSM (methylsulfonylmethane)** is a great source of sulfur, an integral component of the amino acids that are the building blocks of hair protein. MSM improves the strength, sheen and health of hair. In one study, 21 adults (16 men and five women) who were assessed by a certified cosmetologist under the direction of a medical doctor were given MSM or a placebo and then were reassessed at the end of six weeks. The participants did not know who was given MSM and who was given a placebo.

Those given MSM showed significant improvement in hair health, while those taking a placebo showed few or no changes. I recommend a 3,000-mg daily dose of MSM. Look for Opti-MSM or Lignisul MSM, available from many manufacturers and at health-food stores.

•**Essential fatty acids** keep hair from becoming dry and lifeless by decreasing inflammation.

Inflammation worsens the quality of hair folli-cles, and essential fatty acids are needed for the proper development of hair. Food sources include walnuts, eggs, fish, olive oil, flaxseed and hempseed and flax oils. Or you can take a formula like Udo's 3-6-9 Oil Blend, produced by Flora (800-446-2110, *www.florahealth.com*). Follow directions on the label. The formula contains both omega-3 fatty acids (from flax oil or fish oil) and omega-6 fatty acids from evening primrose oil or borage oil. Don't expect immediate results, however. It can take four to six weeks to see improvement.

What Relief! Natural Ways To Curb Your Pain

Not long ago, a 60-year-old woman came to my office suffering from severe arthritis pain in both hands. I gave her a bean-sized dab of a homeopathic gel that she applied directly to the skin on her hands. After a few applications in the span of 30 minutes, her pain was reduced by 90%. She did not need to apply the gel again for two weeks.

I witnessed a similar result with a retired National Football League player. He had severe chronic hip pain from past injuries. With one application of the gel, his pain was relieved by 70% for two full days.

The relief that these people experienced has given them each a new lease on life. *But here's the best news*—unlike pharmaceutical pain relievers, which often cause gastrointestinal upset or damage to internal organs, natural therapies can reduce pain without adverse effects.

WHAT ARE YOU TAKING FOR PAIN?

Most Americans take too many pharmaceutical pain relievers. An estimated 175 million American adults take over-the-counter (OTC) pain relievers regularly. About one-fifth of Americans in their 60s take at least one painkiller for chronic pain on a regular basis.

There has been a lot of news about the life-threatening risks of anti-inflammatory medications such as *rofecoxib* (Vioxx) and *celecoxib* (Celebrex), two pain relievers that had been heavily prescribed by conventional doctors to treat the chronic pain of arthritis and similar conditions. Vioxx was pulled off the market by its manufacturer, Merck, following research that linked it to increased risk of heart attack and stroke. Celebrex now carries warnings about adverse effects, such as increased risk of cardiovascular thrombotic events, heart attack and stroke. Abdominal pain, diarrhea and edema (water retention) may also occur.

Of course, pain-relieving drugs can be a blessing in the event of injury, severe acute migraines or diseases, such as terminal cancer. A number of years ago, when I had a wisdom tooth extracted, I received a local anesthetic. Afterward, I went to an acupuncturist for pain relief so I wouldn't need any painkillers. For about one hour after the acupuncture, I was fine—but then the pain-relieving endorphins wore off. I tried a few natural remedies, but when the pain became excruciating, I resorted to the OTC pain reliever *acetaminophen* (Tylenol). That did the trick.

But many people use painkillers on a regular basis for several months or even years, which increases the risk of dangerous side effects. For instance, people who rely on acetaminophen increase their risk of developing stomach ulcers, liver disease and kidney disease. If you regularly take Celebrex or an OTC nonsteroidal anti-inflammatory drug (NSAID), such as aspirin or *naproxen* (Aleve), you run the risk of kidney and stomach damage. Regular use of NSAIDs also increases risk of heart attack, according to the FDA.

BETTER RESULTS, FEWER RISKS

Before you take any remedy, it's important for your doctor to identify what is causing your pain. Remember, pain is your body's distress signal that something is being irritated or damaged. Sometimes we protect ourselves by reacting instinctively. If you touch something hot, for example, you eliminate the pain by quickly pulling back your hand.

But what if your back hurts? You may need a pain reliever—but back pain also can be a signal that you're harming your body by bending or sitting the wrong way. You may need to address the underlying cause to prevent further injury. Pain receptors are found in the skin, around bones and joints—even in the walls of arteries.

If a muscle is torn, for example, a pain signal is released from fibers in the shredded tissue.

In light of the dangers from prescription and OTC drugs, what safe alternatives are available to you? There are many natural supplements that I recommend.

NATURE'S PAIN RELIEVERS

If you take prescription or OTC pain medication, work with a naturopathic physician, holistic medical doctor or chiropractor who will incorporate natural pain fighters into your treatment regimen. With his/her help, you may be able to reduce your dosage of pain medication (natural pain relievers can be used safely with prescription or OTC painkillers)—or even eliminate the drugs altogether.

Natural pain-fighting supplements are even more effective when combined with physical therapies, such as acupuncture, chiropractic, magnet therapy or osteopathic manipulation (a technique in which an osteopathic physician uses his hands to move a patient's muscles and joints with stretching, gentle pressure and resistance). Physiotherapy (treatment that uses physical agents, such as exercise and massage, to develop, maintain and restore movement and functional ability) also is helpful.

Here are—in no special order—the best natural pain relievers, which can be taken alone or in combination...

•**White willow bark extract** is great for headaches, arthritis, muscle aches and fever. In Europe, doctors prescribe this herbal remedy for back pain, and recent research supports this use. One study conducted in Haifa, Israel, involved 191 patients with chronic low-back pain who took one of two doses of willow bark extract or a placebo daily for four weeks. Researchers found that 39% of patients taking the higher dose of willow bark extract had complete pain relief, compared with only 6% of those taking a placebo. The participants who benefited the most took willow bark extract that contained 240 mg of the compound *salicin*, the active constituent in this herbal remedy. (Aspirin is made from *acetylsalicylic acid*, which has many of the chemical properties of salicin.) However, aspirin can cause gastrointestinal ulceration and other side effects, including kidney damage. Willow bark

extract is believed to work by inhibiting naturally occurring enzymes that cause inflammation and pain.

I recommend taking willow bark extract that contains 240 mg of salicin daily. In rare cases, willow bark extract can cause mild stomach upset. Don't take willow bark if you have a history of ulcers, gastritis or kidney disease. It also should not be taken by anyone who is allergic to aspirin. As with aspirin, willow bark extract should never be given to children under age 12 who have a fever—in rare instances, it can cause a fatal disease called *Reye's syndrome*. Willow bark extract has blood-thinning properties, so avoid it if you take a blood thinner, such as *warfarin* (Coumadin). For low-back pain, you may need to take willow bark extract for a week or more before you get results.

•**Methylsulfonylmethane (MSM)** is a popular nutritional supplement that relieves muscle and joint pain. According to Stanley Jacob, MD, a professor at Oregon Health & Science University who has conducted much of the original research on MSM, this supplement reduces inflammation by improving blood flow. Your cells have receptors that send out pain signals when they're deprived of blood. That's why increased blood flow diminishes pain.

MSM, a natural compound found in green vegetables, fruits and grains, reduces muscle spasms and softens painful scar tissue from previous injuries. A double-blind study of 50 people with osteoarthritis of the knee found that MSM helps relieve arthritis pain.

Start with a daily dose of 3,000 mg to 5,000 mg of MSM. If your pain and/or inflammation doesn't improve within five days, increase the dose up to 8,000 mg daily, taken in several doses throughout the day. If you develop digestive upset or loose stools, reduce the dosage. If you prefer, you can apply MSM cream (per the label instructions) to your skin at the painful area. This product is available at health-food stores and works well for localized pain. MSM has a mild blood-thinning effect, so check with your doctor if you take a blood thinner.

•**S-adenosylmethionine (SAMe)** is a natural compound found in the body. The supplement is an effective treatment for people who have osteoarthritis accompanied by cartilage degeneration. SAMe's ability to reduce pain, stiffness and swelling is similar to that of NSAIDs such as ibuprofen and naproxen, and the anti-inflammatory medication Celebrex. There's also evidence that SAMe stimulates cartilage repair, which helps prevent bones from rubbing against one another. A 16-week study conducted at the University of California, Irvine, compared two groups of people who were being treated for knee pain caused by osteoarthritis. Some took 1,200 mg of SAMe daily, while others took 200 mg of Celebrex. It took longer for people to get relief from SAMe, but by the second month, SAMe proved to be just as effective as Celebrex.

Most patients with osteoarthritis and fibromyalgia (a disorder characterized by widespread pain in muscles, tendons and ligaments) who take SAMe notice improvement within four to eight weeks. Many studies use 1,200 mg of SAMe daily in divided doses. In my experience, taking 400 mg twice daily works well. It's a good idea to take a multivitamin or 50-mg B-complex supplement daily while you're taking SAMe. The vitamin B-12 and folic acid contained in either supplement help your body metabolize SAMe, which means that the remedy goes to work faster.

●**Kaprex** is effective for mild pain caused by injury or osteoarthritis. It is a blend of hops, rosemary extract and *oleanic acid*, which is derived from olive leaf extract. Rather than blocking the body's pain-causing enzymes, these natural substances inhibit pain-causing chemicals called *prostaglandins.*

In a study sponsored by the Institute for Functional Medicine, the research arm of the supplement manufacturer Metagenics, taking Kaprex for six weeks reduced minor pain by as much as 72%. I recommend taking one 440-mg tablet three times daily. Kaprex is manufactured by Metagenics (800-692-9400, *www.metagenics. com*), the institute's product branch. The product is sold only in doctors' offices. To find a practitioner in your area who sells Kaprex, call the toll-free number. Kaprex has no known side effects and does not interact with other medications.

●**Proteolytic enzymes,** including *bromelain, trypsin, chymotrypsin, pancreatin, papain* and a range of protein-digesting enzymes derived from the fermentation of fungus, reduce pain and inflammation by improving blood flow. You can find these natural pain fighters at health-food stores in products labeled "proteolytic enzymes." Take as directed on the label. Bromelain, a favorite of athletes, is available on its own. Extracted from pineapple stems, bromelain reduces swelling by breaking down blood clots that can form as a result of trauma and impede circulation. It works well for bruises, sprains and surgical recovery. If you use bromelain, take 500 mg three times daily between meals.

Repair is a high-potency formula of proteolytic enzymes that I often recommend. It is manufactured by Enzymedica (to find a retailer, call 888-918-1118 or go to *www.enzymedica.com*). Take two capsules two to three times daily between meals. Don't take Repair or any proteolytic enzyme formula if you have an active ulcer or gastritis. Any enzyme product can have a mild blood-thinning effect, so check with your doctor if you take a blood thinner.

●**Pain Med** is the homeopathic gel that gave such quick relief to the patients I described at the beginning of this article. It is remarkably effective for relieving the pain of arthritis, muscle soreness and spasms, sprains, strains, stiffness, headaches (especially due to tension) as well as injuries, including bruises.

Pain Med is a combination of nine highly diluted plant and flower materials, including *arnica, bryonia, hypericum* and *ledum*. Like other homeopathic remedies, it promotes the body's ability to heal itself. A bean-sized dab works well for anyone who has pain. It should be spread on the skin around the affected area. Following an injury, use it every 15 minutes, for a total of up to four applications. As the pain starts to diminish, apply less often. Do not reapply the gel once the pain is gone. Pain Med does not sting, burn or irritate the skin. It is clear, has no odor, does not stain and dries quickly. Because it has so many uses and works so rapidly, Pain Med is a good first-aid remedy to have on hand. To order, contact the manufacturer, GM International, Inc., (800-228-9850, *www.gmipainmed.com*).

Say Good-Bye to Hay Fever

Oh, the sneezing! About 35 million Americans suffer from upper respiratory tract symptoms due to airborne allergies. One of the most common is hay fever, which results from a reaction to pollen.

Pollen enters the nasal cavity and triggers a cascade of reactions that lead to the release of *histamine* and other inflammatory chemicals. This can cause sneezing, coughing and postnasal drip, a runny or congested nose and itchy, watery, red eyes with dark circles underneath. Hay fever can keep you awake at night, making you feel fatigued and generally terrible all day long.

The most widespread pollen allergen is ragweed. One plant can generate a million grains of pollen a day. Other offenders include sagebrush, redroot pigweed, lamb's quarter, Russian thistle (tumbleweed) and English plantain.

Even if none of the plants that cause hay fever are found in your area, you are still susceptible to exposure because the small, light, dry pollen grains are easily transported by wind. Scientists have found ragweed pollen two miles high in the air and up to 400 miles away from its original source.

PREVENTION STRATEGIES

Pollen season occurs during the spring, summer and fall, when pollen is released by trees, grasses and weeds. Pollen counts tend to be highest in the morning, especially on warm, dry, breezy days, and lowest during cool, rainy periods. The pollen concentration is available for most urban areas—check your newspaper. Another resource for pollen counts is the American Academy of Allergy Asthma & Immunology's National Allergy Bureau at *www.aaaai.org/nab*. You can monitor pollen levels and plan accordingly. For example, allergy sufferers should try to stay indoors with the windows closed when pollen levels are high.

You can wear a dust and pollen mask designed to stop pollen from entering the nasal passageways (available at most pharmacies). You can use a high-efficiency particulate air (HEPA) purifier in your house, especially in your bedroom since pollen counts increase during the night.

DRUG THERAPIES

Several pharmaceutical medications can be used to treat hay fever, all of which can have side effects.

We all know about antihistamines, which are used to control excess mucus and reduce itching and sneezing. Examples include the prescription drugs *fexofenadine* (Allegra), *desloratadine* (Clarinex) and *cetirizine* (Zyrtec) and the over-the-counter (OTC) medications *loratadine* (Claritin) and *diphenhydramine* (Benadryl). *Cromolyn sodium* (Nasalcrom) is an OTC nasal spray antihistamine.

Potential side effects of oral medications include drowsiness and impaired coordination. The nasal spray can cause cough, nasal congestion or irritation, nausea, sneezing, throat irritation and wheezing.

Decongestants are used for nasal congestion. A common OTC oral form is *pseudoephedrine* (Sudafed). *Phenylephrine* (NeoSynephrine, Sinex) is a widely used nasal spray. Decongestants may raise blood pressure, cause insomnia and irritability and inhibit urinary flow. They should be avoided by people with high blood pressure and/or glaucoma (they can increase the eye's intraocular pressure). Decongestants should be taken for only a few days—long-term use causes increased blood vessel constriction, which worsens blood pressure.

Corticosteroid treatments contain small doses of steroids to reduce nasal inflammation and swelling. They prevent and treat most allergy symptoms. Common examples of prescription nasal corticosteroids include *fluticasone* (Flonase), *mometasone* (Nasonex) and *triamcinolone* (Nasacort). These nasal corticosteroid sprays can cause fungal infection of the sinuses and mouth.

Sometimes oral steroids are used for severe allergies. These are very powerful prescription medicines that should be used for only a short time (up to a few weeks). Short-term side effects may include weight gain, water retention, high blood pressure, mood swings and depression. Long-term side effects include increased risk for diabetes, cataracts, osteoporosis and muscle weakness.

I know firsthand the miseries of hay fever. Fortunately, the natural approaches I describe below have worked extremely well for me *and* for my patients...

NASAL RINSE

An effective technique for people prone to hay fever and/or sinusitis is nasal irrigation. This involves rinsing the nasal passages with a warm saline solution to reduce the concentration of pollen, dust and other allergens. It also helps to clear excess mucus from the nasal passageways. This is typically done with a neti pot, a small ceramic container with a narrow spout that allows you to pour water into your nostrils and sinus cavities. Neti pots are available at health-food stores for about $20.

To use a neti pot, mix one-quarter teaspoon of salt in a cup of warm water. Pour the solution into the neti pot. Tilt your head to the side, and insert the spout into the upper nostril. The solution will flow into the upper nostril and out the lower nostril. After a few seconds, remove the pot. With your head still tilted, blow through both nostrils. Do not cover one side of your nose—this will force the mucus and bacteria up into your sinuses. Repeat the rinse on the other side. It's messy, but it works. Use once daily for low-grade allergies and twice daily for acute allergies.

An easier alternative is Sinus Rinse. You open a packet of premeasured saline and baking soda, pour it into the bottle that comes with the kit and add warm water. Push the tip of the bottle into one nostril, and squeeze the bottle so the solution comes out the other nostril. Repeat with the other nostril. Do this once or twice daily. A kit containing 50 premixed packets is available from Allergy Solutions for $12.95 (800-491-4300, *www.allergysolution.com*).

Important: To avoid introducing bacteria into your nasal passageways, clean the tip of the neti pot (or Sinus Rinse bottle) with alcohol between uses.

HOMEOPATHIC HELP

Homeopathy treats hay fever by desensitizing the immune system to the offending pollen(s)—or the symptoms they trigger. This is based on the principle that "like cures like"—that is, substances that cause allergy symptoms can be used in a highly diluted form to alleviate those same symptoms.

For example, ragweed, oak and grasses can be taken as individual remedies or as part of a combination remedy. If you know that you are allergic to ragweed pollen, you can take homeopathic ragweed to minimize your response. An allergist can do skin testing to determine which allergens affect you.

Homeopathic remedies are somewhat similar to conventional allergy shots, in which minute doses of the substances you're allergic to are injected under the skin. The advantage of the homeopathic approach is that it is convenient (it requires dissolving some pellets or a liquid solution under your tongue) and relatively inexpensive ($10 to $20 a month).

Researchers at the Southwest College of Naturopathic Medicine and Health Sciences in Tempe, Arizona, conducted a four-week, double-blind clinical trial comparing homeopathic preparations with a placebo during the regional allergy season from February to May. Participants included 40 men and women, ages 26 to 63, diagnosed with moderate to severe seasonal allergy symptoms. Those taking the homeopathic preparations had a 38% reduction in symptoms, such as watery eyes and sneezing, compared with a 26% decline for those using the placebo.

There are two homeopathic remedies that I recommend for the treatment of hay fever. Which one you take depends on your symptoms. They are available at most health-food stores. The dosage is two pellets of a 30C potency twice daily.

•**Allium cepa** (from onion) is for those with watery and burning eyes...runny nose...headache...sneezing.

•**Euphrasia** (from the eyebright plant) is for hay fever that mainly affects only the eyes, causing burning, tearing and redness.

If you don't know which homeopathic remedy to use, try Sabadil Allergy by Boiron, available at health-food stores for about $9. This formula contains six remedies commonly used for hay fever. The typical dose is two tablets dissolved in the mouth every 15 minutes for one hour, then two pellets three times daily.

CHOOSING SUPPLEMENTS

The right supplements also help control hay fever. *My recommendations...*

•**Quercetin,** a type of plant pigment known as a flavonoid, is nature's antihistamine, with anti-inflammatory and antioxidant properties. It is found in onions, apples and green tea. It works best at a starting dosage of 1,000 mg three times daily for five days, followed by a maintenance dosage of 500 mg two or three times daily. Quercetin is very safe, and side effects are uncommon. Quercetin also works well when combined with vitamin C, which may help reduce allergy symptoms in some individuals. A typical dose for hay fever is 3,000 mg to 5,000 mg of vitamin C daily. Reduce the dosage if you develop loose stools. If you have a history of kidney stones, consult your doctor before taking vitamin C supplements.

•**Stinging nettle leaf** is a popular herbal treatment for the relief of hay fever. I have seen it help some patients when used at the first sign of hay fever symptoms. A randomized, double-blind study conducted at the National College of Naturopathic Medicine in Portland, Oregon, involved 69 people with hay fever who took 300 mg of a stinging nettle leaf supplement or a placebo daily. Researchers found that after one week, 58% of those who took stinging nettle leaf had a reduction in symptoms, such as sneezing and itchy eyes, compared with 37% of those who received a placebo.

Interestingly, nettle leaves are a natural source of vitamin C and quercetin. Stinging nettle leaf supplements should be avoided by those with kidney disease because they have a diuretic (water-excreting) effect. The type of stinging nettle leaf used in the study mentioned above is available from Eclectic Institute and can be found at health-food stores.

•**N-acetylcysteine** (NAC) is a great supplement to use if you are suffering from postnasal drip or coughing as the result of mucous formation. I find that 500 mg twice daily is helpful for patients. Side effects, such as nausea, constipation and diarrhea, are rare.

GETTING STARTED

When using homeopathic remedies and supplements, it's best to start two weeks before allergy season and then continue until the end of the season if the treatment is helping. Try quercetin first. If you do not get relief within one week, try stinging nettle leaf, NAC and/or a homeopathic treatment.

A book that I especially like is *Sinus Survival: A Self-Help Guide*, by Robert Ivker, DO (Tarcher).

Put Away Those Dangerous Drugs... And Try These Natural Alternatives

Isn't it strange when some wholesome-looking actor appears on a TV commercial to promote a pharmaceutical? The ad tells you how great the drug is, then proceeds with a long, rapid-fire list of potential side effects. What a contradiction!

It's hard to believe, but Americans spend close to $200 billion each year on prescription drugs. Now, many people are concerned about the side effects of these medications—and with good reason. Each year, 2.9% to 3.7% of hospitalizations in the US are due to adverse reactions to medications.

The solution is to get healthy—and stay healthy—using natural methods. Many nutritional supplements can be used safely and effectively in place of prescription medications. Whether you're treating heartburn, high blood pressure, elevated cholesterol, depression or any number of other common ailments, there are excellent natural alternatives to be considered.

Caution: Do *not* stop taking a prescription drug or begin using a supplement unless you are being monitored by a health professional. These natural alternatives work best when combined with diet and lifestyle improvements, particularly regular exercise, stress-reduction techniques and adequate sleep.

STOMACH MEDICATIONS

Up to 18% of Americans experience heartburn at least once weekly. Heartburn that occurs more than twice a week may be gastroesophageal reflux disease (GERD), a condition in which stomach contents back up into the esophagus. The most commonly prescribed drugs for heartburn and GERD are *esomeprazole* (Nexium), *lansoprazole* (Prevacid), *rabeprazole* (Aciphex), *omeprazole* (Prilosec) and *pantoprazole* (Protonix). Known as proton pump inhibitors (PPIs), these drugs block the production of stomach acid. And they carry a hefty price tag—about $4 per dose. Potential side effects include diarrhea, vomiting, headache, rash, dizziness, abnormal heartbeat, muscle pain, leg cramps and water retention.

Natural alternatives: Try them in this order—each one alone—for two weeks at a time until you find what works effectively for you. You can take more than one at a time.

•**Licorice root** (in chewable wafers or powder form) reduces heartburn and irritation of the digestive tract lining. Take 500 mg to 1,000 mg three times daily 30 minutes before meals. A special type of licorice root, known as *deglycyrrhizinated licorice* (DGL), does not elevate blood pressure, as do some varieties of the herb. DGL is widely available at health-food stores and pharmacies. It should relieve your symptoms within two weeks. Take as needed if symptoms recur.

•**Nux vomica,** a homeopathic remedy derived from the seeds of the poison nut tree, has helped many of my patients reduce or eliminate heartburn. It soothes irritation of the digestive lining and is believed to help the upper esophageal valve close more efficiently, thereby preventing reflux. Take two 30C potency pellets three times daily until your symptoms are eliminated. Improvement should occur within two weeks. Resume treatment if symptoms return. Because nux vomica is also used to treat asthma, it is good for asthmatics who suffer from heartburn.

•**Aloe vera,** a cactuslike member of the lily family, soothes and promotes healing of the lining of the digestive tract. Some people who don't respond to DGL get relief from aloe vera. Drink one-quarter cup of aloe vera juice or take a 500-mg capsule three times daily.

ANTIDEPRESSANTS

Sertaline (Zoloft), *escitalopram* (Lexapro) and *fluoxetine* (Prozac) are the most popular prescription antidepressants sold in the US. They belong to a class of drugs called selective serotonin reuptake inhibitors (SSRIs). *Serotonin,* a neurotransmitter (chemical messenger) produced by nerve cells in the brain, plays an important role in balancing mood. SSRIs temporarily block serotonin from returning to the neuron that released it, boosting the amount of available serotonin.

Potential side effects of SSRIs include drowsiness, nervousness, insomnia, dizziness, nausea, tremors, loss of appetite, headache, diarrhea, dry mouth, irregular heartbeat, skin rash, weight loss or weight gain and activation of mania in patients with bipolar disorder (also known as manic-depressive illness). These drugs also can cause sexual side effects, including loss of libido and decrease in the intensity of orgasms. In July 2005, the FDA warned that children and adults taking antidepressants should be monitored for signs of worsening depression or suicidal thoughts.

Natural alternatives: Try them in this order for six to eight weeks. If effective, continue indefinitely. You can take more than one at a time.

•**S-adenosylmethionine** (SAMe), a nutritional supplement derived from the amino acid *methionine*, is excellent for mild to moderate depression. SAMe is thought to work by increasing the production of mood-boosting neurotransmitters. Some studies have shown SAMe to be as effective as pharmaceutical antidepressants—or, in some cases, even more so. Take 400 mg two or three times daily on an empty stomach. Do not use this supplement if you are taking an antidepressant or antianxiety medication—or if you have bipolar disorder. Like SSRIs, SAMe may activate a manic phase in bipolar patients.

•**5-hydroxytryptophan** (5-HTP) is a quick-acting, mood-enhancing amino acid that I recommend for my patients with mild to moderate depression. In the body, 5-HTP is converted into serotonin, helping to raise levels of this mood-balancing neurotransmitter. Take 100 mg two to three times daily on an empty stomach. Do not take 5-HTP in combination with pharmaceutical antidepressant or antianxiety medication.

•**St. John's wort** is an herb that is widely used in Europe to treat depression. In a review of 23 studies, it was found to be as effective as pharmaceutical therapy for mild to moderate depression. I recommend taking 600 mg of a 0.3% hypericin extract in the morning and 300 mg in the afternoon or evening. St. John's wort should not be used by women who take birth control pills or by anyone taking HIV medication or immune-suppressing drugs. Do not take St. John's wort with antidepressant or antianxiety medication.

• **Fish oil** has been shown to help mild to moderate depression. Take a formula that contains 1,000 mg of combined *docosahexaenoic acid* (DHA) and *eicosapentaenoic acid* (EPA) daily. Nordic Naturals and Carlson's both make good formulas that are available at health-food stores. Fish oil can be taken indefinitely.

• **B vitamins** improve the efficiency of many functions, including the conversion of glucose to fuel and the synthesis of neurotransmitters. Deficiencies of B vitamins (notably B-3) can lead to anxiety and agitation. Take a 50-mg B complex daily for as long as you like.

CHOLESTEROL-LOWERING DRUGS

An estimated 11 million Americans take cholesterol-lowering statins. *Atorvastatin* (Lipitor), *simvastatin* (Zocor) and *rosuvastatin* (Crestor) are the most commonly prescribed in the US. One month's supply of one of these drugs costs $80 to more than $120.

Such drugs work by inhibiting a liver enzyme that helps produce the "bad" cholesterol, known as low-density lipoprotein (LDL) cholesterol. These drugs also decrease fats in the blood known as triglycerides and increase "good" high-density lipoprotein (HDL) cholesterol levels. Possible side effects include abdominal pain and digestive upset, joint pain, and muscle weakness and pain. One of the most frightening side effects is *rhabdomyolysis*. This condition affects only one in 100,000 people taking statins each year, but it results in severe pain and may cause kidney failure.

Natural alternatives: Try red yeast rice extract, then retest cholesterol levels in three months. Continue if effective. If not, try policosanol.

• **Red yeast rice extract** is a supplement that has been shown to reduce total and LDL cholesterol levels by 11% to 32% and triglyceride levels by 12% to 19%. It has been shown to raise HDL by 15% to 30%. Take 2,400 mg of red yeast rice extract (containing 9.6 mg to 13.5 mg total *monacolins*) daily. Side effects, such as mild gastrointestinal discomfort, are rare. As with many products, red yeast rice extract should be avoided by people with liver disease.

Policosanol, a derivative of sugarcane, is another well-researched cholesterol-lowering supplement. The *American Heart Journal* published a review of placebo-controlled studies, which found that taking 10 mg to 20 mg of policosanol daily lowered total cholesterol by 17% to 21% and LDL cholesterol by 21% to 29%. The supplement raised HDL cholesterol by 8% to 15%. Policosanol does not effectively lower triglyceride levels, so I don't recommend it for people who need to reduce these blood fats. Anyone else with high cholesterol should consider taking 10 mg to 20 mg daily.

Important: If your cholesterol levels are significantly elevated (in the mid-300s or higher), you may need to take a statin before trying these natural alternatives. Statins also may be prescribed to help reduce inflammation following a heart attack.

BLOOD PRESSURE MEDICATION

High blood pressure (hypertension) is estimated to affect one of every four adult Americans. *Tenormin* (Atenolol), *lisinopril* (Zestril) and *furosemide* (Lasix) are the most popular prescription drugs for high blood pressure. These drugs are relatively inexpensive—ranging from $11 to $36 per month.

Tenormin (a so-called beta-blocker) works by blocking nerve impulses of the sympathetic nervous system, a portion of the involuntary nervous system that helps control the body's response to stress (the "fight or flight" reaction). Blood pressure is then lowered by reducing the heart rate and the force of the heart muscle contraction. Possible side effects include digestive upset, fatigue, insomnia, impotence, light-headedness, slow heart rate, low blood pressure (a dangerous condition that can lead to fainting and fatigue), numbness, tingling, sore throat and shortness of breath.

Lisinopril is an angiotensin-converting enzyme (ACE) inhibitor. It triggers the relaxation of blood vessels. Relaxed blood vessels help lower blood pressure. Side effects of lisinopril can include chest pain, cough, diarrhea and low blood pressure.

Furosemide is a diuretic that causes water excretion. By blocking absorption of salt and fluid in the kidneys, the drug causes an increase in urine output. Water excretion helps reduce blood volume, which means less work for your arteries and veins. Potential side effects include irregular heartbeat, dizziness, abdominal pain or diarrhea, low blood pressure and an imbalance of electrolytes (key minerals that are needed for vital body functions), leading to muscle cramps or weakness.

Important: If you have moderate to severe high blood pressure (160/100 and above), you may need prescription medication. You may be able to limit your need for prescription blood pressure drugs if you work with your doctor to incorporate natural therapies.

Natural alternatives: Try the first two extracts below for 30 days. If your blood pressure doesn't improve, try using all of the natural treatments together. You should see improvement within four weeks—and can continue the regimen indefinitely.

• **Hawthorn extract,** derived from the berry of a thorny shrub with white or pink flowers, dilates artery walls, decreasing systolic (top number) and diastolic (bottom number) blood pressure by about 10 points each. Take 250 mg to 500 mg three times daily. Hawthorn extract can have a mild blood-thinning effect, so check with your doctor first if you are taking a blood thinner, such as *warfarin* (Coumadin).

• **Bonito fish extract,** a protein from the muscle tissue of the bonito fish, acts like a natural ACE inhibitor. I recommend a daily dose of 1,500 mg.

• **Coenzyme Q10,** an enzyme found in the energy-producing mitochondria of all cells, has been shown to reduce both systolic and diastolic blood pressure by five to 10 points. You may need to take 200 mg to 300 mg daily for a blood pressure–lowering effect.

• **Calcium and magnesium** relax the nervous system and arteries, lowering blood pressure. I suggest 500 mg of calcium and 250 mg of magnesium twice daily.

Save Your Eyesight ... With the Right Foods And Supplements

Vision is an amazing gift. The nutrients we absorb from our food enhance and maintain circulation to keep the tissues and structures in our eyes healthy. Without proper nutrition and eye protection, we run the risk of developing eye disease.

Cataracts and age-related macular degeneration affect about 29 million Americans age 40 and older. Both can lead to partial vision loss or blindness.

Cataracts develop slowly, causing a clouding of the eye lens that impairs vision. About half of all Americans over age 65 have some degree of cataract formation. Cataract surgery has a high success rate, but it's better to prevent cataracts from forming in the first place.

Macular degeneration is more serious. It occurs when the macula (the part of the eye that allows us to see detail in the center of our vision field) becomes damaged and deteriorates. This leads to the loss of central vision and makes it difficult to read and see small objects, such as buttons on a cuff.

The two main types of macular degeneration are dry and wet. The dry type accounts for about 85% of cases and can be prevented and treated with proper nutrition. The wet type is caused by abnormal blood vessel growth under the retina (the light-sensitive layer lining the interior of the eye). Laser treatments can improve this type but won't cure it.

To help prevent eye disease, you must avoid the formation of free radicals. These harmful molecules come from a variety of sources, including exposure to smoke (from tobacco, fireplaces, etc.) and toxic metals, such as lead, which are found in some water supplies, as well as from fried foods.

In addition, it is crucial to wear sunglasses that block 100% of ultraviolet A (UVA) and ultraviolet B (UVB) rays. UVA rays are associated with the development of macular degeneration, while UVB rays are linked to the formation of cataracts. Not all sunglasses block both types of rays, so read the label carefully to find a pair that does. Wear them anytime you're out in the sun. If you already have cataracts or macular degeneration, wear sunglasses whenever you're outside during daytime, even when it is overcast.

Best choice: Wraparound sunglasses, which prevent damaging rays from entering from the sides.

EYE-PROTECTING NUTRIENTS

A number of nutrients can help you prevent— and even treat—cataracts and macular degeneration. Although fresh foods are the best source of most eye-protecting nutrients, supplements help ensure that you're getting adequate amounts. If you already have been diagnosed with one of these eye conditions, you should be taking supplements, even if you are undergoing conventional treatment. Adults who are concerned about developing eye disease also should consider taking eye-protecting supplements.

Each nutrient listed below can be purchased individually or as part of a vision formula. Individual supplements typically provide higher dosages, but people who don't like to bother with a lot of bottles may prefer a vision formula that combines many key nutrients. Good eye formulas include Vision Optimizer by Jarrow Formulas (to find a retailer in your area, call 800-726-0886 or go to *www.jarrow.com*) and Visual Eyes Multinutrient Complex by Source Naturals (to find a retailer in your area, call 800-815-2333 or go to *www.sourcenaturals.com*).

The most important eye-protecting nutrients…

•**Lutein** is part of the carotenoid family (fat-soluble pigments found in plants). This antioxidant helps filter all types of light, including UV rays, that damage cells of the eye, particularly the macula. Population studies have found an association between a high dietary intake of lutein and a decreased risk of developing macular degeneration and cataracts.

Lutein-rich foods: Egg yolks, spinach, broccoli, kale and corn. Most Americans get only 1 mg to 2 mg of lutein in their daily diets, but eye-disease prevention requires higher levels of this nutrient. People with macular degeneration or cataracts should take a supplement that contains 15 mg of lutein daily. To prevent these diseases, take 2 mg to 5 mg of lutein daily as part of a high-potency multivitamin or eye formula. Because lutein is fat soluble, it should be taken with a meal for best absorption. Lutein has no known side effects.

•**Zeaxanthin** also is in the carotenoid family. Like lutein, zeaxanthin protects the eye from the damaging effects of UV rays. Zeaxanthin is found in the same foods as lutein, as well as oranges and tangerines. Supplemental eye formulas and mixed carotenoid complexes contain zeaxanthin. People with macular degeneration should take a supplement that contains 3 mg of zeaxanthin daily with a meal. For prevention, take 500 micrograms (mcg) to 1 mg daily. There are no known side effects.

•**Vitamin C** protects against cataracts and macular degeneration. As people age, vitamin C levels in the eye decrease. That's why it is so important to eat foods that are rich in vitamin C and take a supplement that contains this nutrient. Population studies have found that people taking multivitamins or any supplements containing vitamins C and E for more than 10 years had a 60% lower risk of developing cataracts. To prevent cataracts and macular degeneration, take 500 mg of vitamin C daily. People who already have eye disease, especially cataracts, should take 2,000 mg to 3,000 mg daily in divided doses.

Note: If you experience loose stools from this dose, reduce your intake by 500 mg daily until symptoms subside. People with a history of kidney stones should check with a doctor before taking high-dose vitamin C.

•**Bilberry** contains antioxidant complexes known as *anthocyanidins*. These phytonutrients protect the lens and other eye tissue against the free radical damage associated with cataracts and macular degeneration. People who have cataracts or macular degeneration should take 160 mg two to three times daily of a 25% anthocyanoside extract. Take the same dose for prevention. Bilberry has no significant side effects.

•**Vitamin E complex,** taken at a dose of 400 international units (IU) with 80 mg of zinc, 500 mg of vitamin C and 15 mg of beta-carotene daily, has been shown to reduce the risk of visual acuity loss by 27% and curb by 25% the risk for progression of macular degeneration in people with an advanced form of this disease. Researchers have estimated that 300,000 of the 8 million Americans with macular degeneration (in one or both eyes) could prevent their eye disease from advancing and avoid any associated vision loss during the next five years by taking this supplement combination. For eye-disease prevention, take 200 IU of a mixed vitamin E complex that contains the vitamin E subgroups *tocopherols* and *tocotrienols*. People diagnosed with macular degeneration or cataracts should take 400 IU of a mixed vitamin E complex daily, along with the other nutrients listed in this section.

•**Zinc** promotes the activity of enzymes in the retina. When used alone or in combination with other antioxidants, such as beta-carotene, vitamin C or vitamin E, zinc has been shown to reduce the risk of vision loss associated with macular degeneration. If you have cataracts or macular degeneration, take 45 mg to 80 mg of zinc daily, along with 1 mg to 2 mg of copper (zinc supplements can lower copper levels in the body). For prevention, take 15 mg to 30 mg of zinc daily and 1 mg to 2 mg of copper. Side effects, such as occasional digestive upset, are rare.

•**Betaine hydrochloride (betaine HCl)** supports healthy digestion and absorption. Not only do many older adults not consume enough fruits and vegetables to get ample nutrition for their eyes, but their digestion is too poor to make good use of what they do eat. Stomach acid levels are believed to decrease as people age, which can hinder mineral absorption from foods and supplements. Betaine HCl mimics the *hydrochloric acid* normally produced by the stomach. I highly recommend that anyone with cataracts or macular degeneration take one or two 500-mg or 600-mg capsules of betaine HCl with each meal. Use the same dose to help prevent eye disease. People taking antacid medications and those with reflux disease or active ulcers should not use betaine HCl because it can aggravate these conditions.

•**B vitamins,** such as vitamin B-1 (*thiamine*), vitamin B-2 (*riboflavin*) and vitamin B-3 (*niacin*), are associated with a decreased risk of cataracts when consumed at high levels. These B vitamins, especially riboflavin and niacin, are believed to help regenerate *glutathione*, a powerful antioxidant found in the body's cells, including the eye lens. Most high-potency multivitamins contain these B vitamins in adequate amounts (2 mg of B-1, 3 mg of B-2 and 40 mg of B-3) to help prevent eye disease. For people diagnosed with cataracts, take an additional 50-mg B complex daily.

•**N-acetylcarnosine** has recently received a great deal of attention from nutrition-oriented doctors as a treatment for cataracts. Its parent compound, *L-carnosine*, is a molecule composed of the two amino acids *histidine* and *alanine*. N-acetylcarnosine acts as an antioxidant and has been shown to protect cell membranes from oxidative damage. A 2001 Russian study involving two randomized, double-blind, placebo-controlled trials found that N-acetylcarnosine eyedrops improved visual acuity and glare sensitivity in 26 of 41 cataract patients (average age 65). The dose used in this study was two drops twice daily of a 1% aqueous solution. The same type of eyedrops used in the study are available for $39.95 in a product called Can-C, manufactured by Smart Nutrition (858-270-7907, *www. smart-nutrition.net*). Cataract patients who use these drops should be monitored by a doctor.

INTRAVENOUS THERAPY

The most aggressive natural therapy for people with macular degeneration is intravenous (IV) therapy, which involves the infusion of nutrients in a solution directly into the bloodstream via a needle inserted into a vein in the arm. This method provides a much greater therapeutic dose of nutrients to the cells of the macula, since it bypasses the digestive tract.

Jonathan Kalman, ND, who practices at my clinic, specializes in IV therapy for serious diseases. He routinely administers IV nutrients such as glutathione, zinc, vitamin C, B vitamins and mineral complexes. In many cases, this type of treatment can halt the progression of the dry form of macular degeneration and often improves vision. Dr. Kalman recommends an initial series of 15 twice-weekly treatments. To find a doctor who offers IV therapy, consult the American College for Advancement in Medicine (800-532-3688, *www.acamnet.org*). IV therapy costs $100 to $125 per treatment. It's not covered by insurance, but it can be well worth the investment.

EYE NUTRIENTS

Here is a summary of my recommendations for people diagnosed with eye disease. Preventive doses appear in parentheses.

CATARACTS

•**Lutein.** 15 mg daily (2 mg to 5 mg daily in a high-potency multivitamin or eye formula).

•**Vitamin C.** 2,000 mg to 3,000 mg daily (500 mg daily).

•**Bilberry.** 160 mg two to three times daily of a 25% anthocyanoside extract (same dose).

•**Vitamin E complex.** 400 IU daily (200 IU daily).

•**Zinc.** 45 mg to 80 mg daily with 1 mg to 2 mg of copper (15 mg to 30 mg daily with 1 mg to 2 mg of copper).

•**Betaine hydrochloride.** One to two 500- to 600-mg capsules with each meal (same dose).

•**Vitamin B complex.** 50 mg daily plus a high-potency multivitamin (high-potency multivitamin).

•**N-acetylcarnosine eyedrops.** Two drops twice daily of a 1% aqueous solution, used under a doctor's supervision.

MACULAR DEGENERATION

Take the first six supplements listed above, plus…

•**Zeaxanthin.** 3 mg daily (500 mcg to 1 mg daily).

•**Beta-carotene.** 15 mg daily (same dose).

Restless Legs and Sleep Apnea

Restless legs syndrome (RLS) is characterized by an overwhelming urge to move the legs when you are at rest. Usually, this urge is accompanied by abnormal sensations beneath the skin that are best described as uncomfortable crawling, tingling, itching and/or pulling.

RLS may be related to low oxygen levels caused by sleep apnea, a potentially dangerous condition in which you stop breathing for short periods at night without realizing it. Speak with your doctor about sleep apnea treatments. For my patients, I recommend losing weight and wearing dental appliances at night to keep the airway open.

The cause of RLS is unknown. Prescription drugs are commonly used, but I find that the following natural therapies are effective…

•**Vitamin and mineral supplements.** Ask your doctor to check your blood for deficiencies in iron, folic acid and magnesium. Deficiencies in one or more of these nutrients have been shown to contribute to RLS. Once a deficiency

is corrected, RLS symptoms should improve in a few weeks. To relax the muscles and nerves, many of my patients with RLS take 500 mg of calcium citrate or chelate and 250 mg to 500 mg of magnesium each evening.

•**Dietary changes.** RLS can occur when blood sugar drops too low. Eat regular meals throughout the day, and try a protein shake—mix protein powder with soy, almond or rice milk—in the evening for more stable blood sugar levels during the night.

•**Acupuncture.** Consider treatments from a qualified practitioner. Acupuncture normalizes nerve flow and muscle contractions.

Fibrocystic Breast Disease

Forty-four-year-old Pauline suffered from fibrocystic breast disease (FBD), a noncancerous condition characterized by lumpy breasts that are tender or painful. Symptoms often intensify before or during menstruation. This condition affects approximately 60% of all women, commonly between the ages of 30 and 50. Having lived with FBD for years, Pauline was searching for natural approaches to relieve her symptoms. Conventional doctors offered her pain medicine or birth control pills, but neither was a good option in her mind, because they did not address the underlying cause.

I explained to Pauline that most women who have FBD also have a hormone imbalance—specifically, progesterone levels that are lower than what is optimal during the last two weeks of their menstrual cycles. Or I find that their progesterone levels are normal, but estrogen levels are elevated, leading to a high level of estrogen relative to progesterone. Some women also develop FBD as a result of low thyroid function. In Pauline's case, testing showed mildly low levels of thyroid and progesterone hormones. Since these hormone levels were only slightly low, I recommended a thyroid glandular supplement that supports thyroid function. I also prescribed homeopathic Pulsatilla, a great hormone balancer that treats FBD symptoms, including breast tenderness. I often prescribe natural progesterone for the treatment of FBD, since it works so well. But in Pauline's case, I felt the use of nutritional supplements and dietary changes would be all she needed.

As we spoke more, I learned that Pauline sometimes consumed two foods that are associated with FBD due to their caffeine content—coffee and chocolate.

Also high in caffeine: Black tea and colas (diet and regular), as well as some over-the-counter drugs, such as headache and menstrual cramp medications, and some pain relief and cold remedies. Some studies have shown that the complete avoidance of caffeine-containing foods is helpful for FBD. I also recommended the herb chasteberry, which has been shown to relieve premenstrual breast pain. Chasteberry increases progesterone production by the ovaries. When two capsules (240 mg each) are taken every morning, reduced breast pain is usually noted within two to three menstrual cycles.

Finally, I asked Pauline to take fish oil and evening primrose oil—each contains a blend of essential fatty acids, important for reducing inflammation and regulating hormones. Fish oil contains *eicosapentaenoic acid* (EPA), which has anti-inflammatory effects. Evening primrose oil contains *gamma linoleic acid* (GLA), which reduces pain and inflammation. After two months, Pauline reported that her breast tenderness had decreased significantly. When I saw her again four months later, she reported no breast tenderness or swelling. The lumpiness of her breasts was reduced significantly as well.

Antioxidants and Chemotherapy

Many oncologists fear that supplementing with antioxidants (nutrients that neutralize negatively charged molecules called *free radicals*) may diminish the effectiveness of some types of chemotherapy, which work by creating free radicals that destroy cancer cells.

Researchers reviewed 19 studies involving 1,554 subjects who regularly took antioxidant supplements (such as *glutathione, melatonin* and/or vitamins A, C and E).

Results: In 17 trials, patients on chemotherapy who took antioxidants were more likely to survive and/or to have tumors shrink, compared with those in control groups. In eight studies, antioxidant users were less likely to experience chemotherapy side effects severe enough to require dosage reductions.

My view: Antioxidants help the body detoxify during chemotherapy and protect against organ damage—while allowing patients to continue their chemotherapy at optimal doses (due to more tolerable side effects) and also keeping noncancerous cells healthy.

Fish Oil for Heart Disease And More

Gary's father had died at the age of 54. "It was a heart attack," Gary told me.

Now 44 himself, Gary almost felt as if he were living on borrowed time. He could hear the clock ticking.

I assured him that most cases of heart attacks can be prevented. I also let him know he was doing the right thing—showing some concern about his heart health before anything happened. Most people, sad to say, wait until they've had a heart attack before taking the measures that they could and should have taken years before.

True, there are inherited factors that make some people more susceptible than others to heart attack—specifically, homocysteine and cholesterol levels just seem to be higher in some people than in others. But most heart attacks are due to diet and lifestyle factors.

Gary had done enough reading to be aware of that. It was one reason he wanted to get started on an aggressive program to keep his heart as healthy as possible.

Among the strategies we discussed were stress reduction, exercise, a series of lab tests, and, of course, diet and supplements. I emphasized the importance of omega-3 fatty acids found in fish,

especially cold-water fish such as salmon, mackerel, herring and sardines. Above all, I recommended fish-oil supplements, such as salmon oil,
to optimize the amount of these heart-healthy
fatty acids. As part of a total strategy for heart
health, the steady intake of fish oil could, potentially, add decades to his life expectancy.

OIL WELL

Among the essential fatty acids that we need
to live, omega-3s are very important. These are
fats that your body can't manufacture on its own,
so they need to come from food sources or supplements.

While omega-3 is also found in flaxseed and
flaxseed oil, the kind that you get from fish and
fish oil has some unique properties that are not
present in these other foods. The fish and fish
oils are a direct source of two long-chain fatty
acids known as EPA (eicosapentanoic acid) and
DHA (docosahexanoic acid), and both are very
important for heart health.

Another reason doctors are confident about
the benefits of fish oil is pragmatic. The vast
majority of studies on essential fatty acids have
been done on fish oils. There are sound reasons
to believe that oils such as flaxseed oil may be
nearly as effective, but to date, they haven't been
studied so much. It is the fish oils that have been
studied and shown to be effective.

Fish became more popular as a "healthy
heart" food when researchers studied the "Mediterranean diet"—that is, the diet of many cultures
around the Mediterranean during the 1960s in
Crete, parts of Greece and southern Italy. (There,
as in many other cultures, the "American diet"
has crept in, raising the rate of heart disease and
other chronic diseases.) In the classic Mediterranean diet, people had many plant foods (vegetables, legumes, fruit, bread, pasta, nuts), lots of
olive oil, and low to moderate amounts of fish,
poultry, meat, dairy, eggs and wine.

Nutritionists believe the consumption of fish
was one of the key benefits of this diet, which
resulted in a much lower incidence of obesity,
heart disease, diabetes, and cancer. A four-year
study of the Mediterranean diet found that people could reduce their risk of heart attack by as
much as 70 percent.

SEA RATIONS

In a more direct study of fish consumption, a
team of researchers who looked at mortality data
from 36 countries confirmed that life expectancy
is longer in those countries where people get a
lot of fish in their daily diet. Men and women
who eat more fish have a lower risk of early
death from all kinds of illnesses, particularly
stroke and heart disease.

Essential fatty acids form a group of hormone-
like messengers known as prostaglandins. The
omega-3 fatty acids as found in fish oil—helped
along by the EPA and DHA in the fish—tend to
decrease inflammation, thin the blood and balance the immune system.

In the immune system, EPA appears to be particularly important for its anti-inflammatory effects, so it's helpful to people who have arthritis.
DHA is critical for the proper development and
function of the brain because your brain cells
need it to transmit electrical impulses efficiently.
It's not surprising, therefore, that a DHA deficiency can lead to memory, behavior and learning problems.

Some studies have also indicated that supplementing infant formula with DHA can improve
children's IQ. Interestingly, it's also important for
mood regulation, and studies have shown that a
deficiency can contribute to depression.

The DHA found in fish oil also appears to calm
down hyperactive children. It's also required for
proper retinal development for infants.

DOSAGE

Fish oil capsules generally are available in 500-
to 1,000-milligram doses. When purchasing the
capsules, pay particular attention to the amounts
of EPA and DHA stated on the labels. You want
fish oils that contain about 18 percent EPA and
12 percent DHA: in other words, totalling about
30 percent of the omega-3 fatty acids found in
these fish oils. (Some of the newly developed,
high-potency fish oils now contain even higher
concentrations of EPA and DHA.)

For preventative purposes, I recommend that
people eat foods high in DHA and EPA such as
cold-water fish. (Eggs also contain DHA.)

If your health is generally good, I'd advise taking 2,000 milligrams of a daily fish-oil supplement such as salmon oil. But if you're susceptible
to specific diseases such as arthritis, high blood

pressure and other conditions, I'd advise getting a higher dose—as much as 6,000 to 10,000 milligrams per day. However, you'll probably want to check with your health practitioner to find an optimal dose for your condition, since the supplement can be costly.

If you're taking the concentrated fish-oil capsules that have higher concentrations of EPA and DHA, I recommend salmon oil or tuna oil capsules that have been tested for heavy metal contamination and rancidity. I am also a big fan of the oil blends that contain a combination of essential fatty acids such as DHA, EPA, and GLA. An ideal formula also has vitamin E in it. If not, take vitamin E *with* the fish oil to prevent the oil from going rancid.

Fish-oil capsules should be stored in the refrigerator once they are opened. Don't leave the container standing in bright light or keep it in a warm room.

WHAT ARE THE SIDE EFFECTS?

Some people who take fish oil experience digestive upset including burping—which can be disconcerting because you may burp a "fishy" smell. But you probably won't have that problem if you take the capsules with meals.

Also, some companies make specially designed capsules that ensure the oil makes it into the small intestine before breaking down. Such claims are advertised so you might want to try their capsules to see whether their product alleviates the problem of burping or "fish breath."

Since fish oils also have a blood-thinning effect, check with your doctor if you are taking any blood-thinning medications.

You may have an increase in LDL cholesterol while supplementing fish oil. If a blood test shows your cholesterol count is on the rise, you can take a garlic supplement to help neutralize this potential effect of the fish oil.

Although people have relatively few and minor problems with the side effects of fish oil, there's a risk that the capsules can contain rancid oil. It's easy to check, however. Just cut open the end of a capsule. If the fish oil has gone rancid, you can easily smell the strong odor. You're better off getting a fresh bottle with new capsules.

Finally, check the label of any brand you buy to make sure the product was tested for contaminants such as heavy metals.

Here are my fish oil recommendations for various conditions…

ADD AND ADHD

Many school-age children have been diagnosed with Attention Deficit Disorder (ADD) or Attention Deficit Hyperactivity Disorder (ADHD), and their problems are sometimes related to nutritional imbalances. (Excess sugars and some additives in junk food have particularly been blamed.)

Essential fatty acids such as DHA are critically important for proper brain function, but—well, how many children do you know who eat fresh cold-water fish three times a week? When children aren't getting enough DHA and they're loading up on saturated fat, trans fatty acids and omega-6 fatty acids from fast-foods, the inevitable result is a fatty-acid imbalance.

DHA supplementation has been shown to decrease aggression while a child is under stress. The DHA in fish oil helps to improve the chemical balance in the brain while giving the general benefits of omega 3 fatty acid supplementation.

I recommend that bottle-fed infants receive omega-3 supplementation, especially DHA, for proper brain and retina development. Breast-fed infants receive these critical essential fatty acids in the breast milk. I suspect that, before long, DHA supplementation will be required in all commercial baby formulas.

ARTHRITIS

Numerous studies with fish oil have been done on people with rheumatoid arthritis and the results have been very positive. For aggressive treatment using fish oil, take 6,000 milligrams daily. Some people need doses that are even higher, so talk to your health practitioner about the optimum dose if you have severe rheumatoid arthritis.

If the fish oil is helpful in reducing stiffness and pain, there's a good chance you'll be able to reduce the dosages of pharmaceuticals. Drug therapy for rheumatoid arthritis focuses on prednisone, methotrexate (also used for chemotherapy) and anti-inflammatory medications—all of which can have serious toxicity when used on a long-term basis. With fish oil, on the other hand, there's no toxicity, so it's a far more benign treatment than the classic pharmaceuticals. One study found that many patients were able to go off their anti-inflammatory drugs while supplementing fish oil and experienced no relapse in their rheumatoid arthritis. Researchers found that the fish oil had a balancing effect on the entire immune system.

It is recommended, as the result of studies, that a minimum daily dose of 3,000 milligrams EPA and DHA is necessary to derive the expected benefits, although I find not all my patients need this high a dosage. Once you start taking fish oil, you can expect to stay on it for at least 12 weeks before it begins to yield benefits. But after that, you can stay on it indefinitely.

Despite the many improvements you can get from fish oil, I do have to say it should be part of a total program when you're treating rheumatoid arthritis. It's also important to improve your diet and take steps to reduce the toxins in your body. I've seen the quickest results with detoxification programs when they also involved homeopathic remedies. But fish oil is a good long-term therapy for some people, and it can definitely help keep inflammatory conditions under control.

Although not so well studied, essential fatty acids found in fish oil are helpful to decrease the stiffness associated with osteoarthritis, the most common form of arthritis, where the cartilage has degenerated.

ASTHMA

The rate of asthma keeps increasing. Sadly, children's asthma is continuing to rise at an alarming rate. Environmental pollution and poor dietary habits are largely to blame.

Essential fatty acids in fish and fish oil help to suppress the inflammatory chemicals involved in this disease. Studies show that children who eat oily fish more than once a week have one-third the risk of getting asthma as children who do not eat fish or eat lean fish on a regular basis.

Fish-oil supplements are helpful for both children and adults with asthma. Again, the benefits of fish oil take months before the natural anti-inflammatory benefits begin to take hold.

CANCER

Omega-3 fatty acids are important for a healthy, well-functioning immune system. If you can get more omega-3 fatty acids in your diet and also take supplements, there's a good chance you can help protect yourself from certain types of cancers.

Animal studies have shown that fish oil can augment certain types of chemotherapy to fight cancer more effectively. Fish oil has also been shown to help treat *cachexia,* which is the loss of muscle mass and weight in cancer patients.

CARDIOVASCULAR DISEASE

With many studies to back up its benefits, fish oil is often recommended as a preventative for heart and circulation problems. Along with the population studies showing that consumption of fish oil slashes the rate of cardiovascular disease, are literally hundreds of studies that support these observations. Fish oils reduce cholesterol and triglyceride levels and also act as a natural blood thinner, which results in the lowering of blood pressure.

CHRONIC OBSTRUCTIVE PULMONARY DISEASE

Over 17 million Americans suffer from this group of serious breathing disorders that includes asthma, bronchitis, and emphysema. Smoking, as you might expect is the factor that multiplies your chances of getting any of these diseases. But for smokers as well as nonsmokers, there are some benefits in eating fish as often as possible.

CROHN'S DISEASE AND ULCERATIVE COLITIS

Inflammatory bowel diseases such as Crohn's disease and ulcerative colitis can be helped by fish-oil supplementation.

In one study of ulcerative colitis, people who took fish-oil supplements (high in omega-3's) were able to cut their steroid medications in half. Again, I see fish oil as one component of a total natural-therapy program to address and alleviate these digestive conditions. Other measures include stress reduction, improving digestive capacity and maintaining a healthful diet.

Herbal medicines and homeopathy are excellent therapies to help turn these conditions around without relying on pharmaceutical drugs that may have many damaging side effects.

DEPRESSION

The brain is 60 percent fat and requires essential fatty acids, especially DHA, to function properly. It has been shown that people with deficiency in DHA are much more likely to suffer from depression.

Consuming fish on a regular basis is a good way to prevent depression. I recommend concentrated DHA supplements for those already battling depression.

As a side note, I believe it's time that more research is done on nutritional deficiencies to find out how they can cause mental diseases such as depression. I see an increasing number of people using pharmaceutical antidepressants on a long-term basis, without exploring other preventives. As we learn more about genetic susceptibility to depression, we will also discover what nutrients and other therapies can help correct what people have come to call *genetic depression*. To date, fish oil is certainly one of the most important of the nutrients we have been able to identify as necessary for healthy brain functioning.

ECZEMA

I have found that flaxseeds and flaxseed oil in combination with GLA work well for eczema. It also makes sense to consume cold-water fish rich in omega-3 fatty acids. Fish oil is also another option to treat eczema.

HIGH BLOOD PRESSURE

High blood pressure is one of the biggest risk factors for heart disease and stroke. Numerous studies have shown that fish oil reduces blood pressure. I find fish oil works best as part of a natural program—combined with stress-reduction techniques and a regimen that includes herbs such as hawthorn, minerals such as magnesium and calcium, along with the natural supplement CoQ10.

HIGH TRIGLYCERIDES

With fish oil, you can lower high triglyceride levels, which are an independent risk factor for heart disease. As I've mentioned, though, fish oil can increase LDL cholesterol, so you'll want to supplement with garlic to help balance out its effects.

INSULIN RESISTANCE

The inability to metabolize carbohydrates effectively leads to high blood-sugar levels and a corresponding spike of the hormone insulin (the component that helps get the blood sugar into the cells). As a result, many different biochemical reactions can occur, one of which is weight gain.

Clinical studies have shown that omega-3 fatty acids, such as those in fish oil, help improve the body's utilization of insulin. (It's interesting that an essential fatty acid can help *decrease* body fat!) This insulin-balancing effect is also important in relation to diabetes.

KIDNEY PROTECTION

People who receive organ transplants require extensive immune-suppressing drugs. These are needed to keep the body from rejecting the donated organ, but some of the drugs (such as cyclosporine) are so powerful that they can have life-threatening side effects.

In the case of patients who have had kidney transplants, however, it's been shown that they resume normal kidney function more quickly when omega-3–rich fish oil is supplemented. It appears that the fish oil actually protects the kidneys from the damaging effects of the immune-suppressing drugs.

LUPUS

Two pilot studies have shown fish oil to benefit people with lupus, an autoimmune condition where the immune system attacks its own tissue. For patients with lupus, I suggest eating cold-water fish regularly and supplementing with fish oil. It may take six months to a year before there's any improvement, but sometimes the benefits can be dramatic.

MULTIPLE SCLEROSIS

Dr. Roy Swank, the doctor who developed a natural protocol for multiple sclerosis (MS), recommended fish oil as well as flaxseed oil. In fact, Dr. Swank advocated that patients who have MS should eat fish three times a week or more. He was also a proponent of cod liver oil—one of the popular fish oils—as a daily supplement.

PSORIASIS

Several studies have shown that 10 to 12 grams of fish oil daily can improve psoriasis. I routinely recommend fish oil and dietary fish as well as other natural therapies to improve this inflammatory condition.

SCHIZOPHRENIA

Some preliminary studies are showing that EPA and DHA may be helpful in the treatment of schizophrenia. More research needs to be done, but I would not be surprised to see these essential fatty acids become accepted as part of the routine treatment for schizophrenia. Dr. Abraham Hoffer of Victoria, British Columbia has already demonstrated that a knowledgeable practitioner can provide a full-scale treatment of schizophrenia with nutritional therapies.

Echinacea—The Best-Selling Immune Booster

It's not unusual to get calls at my office from patients wondering what to do about the cold or flu that just hit them. My first thought is: What natural supplements can they get quickly, right off the shelf?

Well, just about anyone can find echinacea (pronounced *eck-in-AY-sha*) at a nearby store. It's one of the five top-selling herbs in North America. In fact, it's a worldwide best-seller, as herbalists and doctors in Europe have been prescribing echinacea for decades. Carrying the popular name of purple coneflower (so-called because of its beautiful, purple, daisylike petals), echinacea is renowned as an herb that enhances the immune system. It's commonly used to treat a number of conditions from flu and the common cold to a range of other infectious diseases.

THE SNAKEBITE CONNECTION

Native Americans of the Plains are believed to be the first to use echinacea. As today, it was a remedy for colds, coughs and sore throats, but also toothaches, battle wounds and even rattlesnake bites.

During the latter part of the 1800s, Plains settlers adopted the purple coneflower as a common remedy; and by the 1920s, echinacea was being sold as a commercial product and prescribed by the many physicians who were comfortable with herbal medicines.

Dr. H.C.F. Meyer of Pawnee, Nebraska, was a keen commercial promoter. Adding his own recommendations to what he had learned from Native Americans, Dr. Meyer sold echinacea as a cure all for various ailments. His reputation was considerably enhanced by the claim that he had successfully treated 613 cases of rattlesnake poisoning. *One doctor gave the following candid account of Dr. Meyer's own, personal echinacea experiment...*

"With the courage of his convictions upon him, he injected the venom of the crotalus (rattlesnake) into the first finger of his left hand; the swelling was rapid and in six hours up to the elbow. At this time he took a dose of the remedy, bathed the part thoroughly, and laid down to pleasant dreams. On awakening in four hours, the pain and swelling were gone."

INFECTION FIGHTER TO THE RESCUE

I can't say I have had any patients come to me for the natural treatment of rattlesnake bites. (If I did, I would quickly hurry them off to a hospital emergency room for a dose of up-to-date antivenom.) But it's interesting to note that echinacea does have the special property of preventing the spread of infectious substances to tissues.

Echinacea as a healing remedy was introduced to Europe during the 1930s. Since then the preponderance of scientific research on echinacea has been done in Western Europe, especially Germany, where the government plays an active role in funding natural-medicine research. But Canadian and American researchers have recently made similar strides in echinacea research, with clinical studies and biochemical analysis of the healing herb.

Over 400 studies to date have looked at the pharmacology and clinical uses of echinacea. Not all studies have shown efficacy of the herb, but most of the research indicates that echinacea helps reinforce the immune system.

Echinacea is consistently one of the best-selling herbs in North America and Europe. Over 10 million units are sold annually in Germany alone.

Though there are nine species of echinacea, *Echinacea purpurea* and *Echinacea angustifolia* are the two most often used commercially. Most clinical studies are done with these species, especially *purpurea*.

TONGUE-TINGLING CHEMICALS

Scientists have not reached a consensus about the active ingredients in echinacea. Though researchers acknowledge the herb has many immune-boosting properties as well as anti-inflammatory and antimicrobial effects, they're not sure what chemicals or combination of chemicals are responsible.

It's known, however, that echinacea contains caffeic acid derivatives such as cichoric acid and polysaccharides. The plant also has compounds known as alkylamides that are thought to be important. (Alkylamides are the substances that make your tongue tingle and go numb if you take a hefty dose of straight echinacea.)

Some of these compounds are water-soluble and some are alcohol-soluble. When tinctures, pills or tablets are being created from echinacea, the manufacturer must go through an elaborate process to extract the compounds. Recent research done at the University of British Columbia in conjunction with the University of Alberta has shown that the ratio of the actives in echinacea is important for optimal immune response. So in other words, not only is it important to have active constituents in echinacea products, but to also have them in a specific ratio or blend.

AROUSING IMMUNE CELLS

Echinacea doesn't work like the pharmaceutical antibiotics that "kill" microbes like bacteria. Instead, echinacea arouses the immune cells that patrol and defend the body against these invaders. It increases the number and activity of disease-fighting white blood cells, and it activates antiviral chemicals such as interferon. Echinacea can even activate the immune cells that fight tumors. In addition, research has shown that the chemicals in echinacea have the power to inhibit an enzyme released by bacteria, called *hyaluronidase*. Bacteria normally produce this enzyme to penetrate into human tissue. Echinacea prevents this from happening.

Researchers in a German study found clear evidence that echinacea helps to promote good immune cells, called *phagocytes*. One group of people were given 30 drops of echinacea three times daily for five days, while people in the control group were given a placebo. The level of phagocytes was measured at the beginning and throughout the study. At day three, the phagocyte activity of those taking echinacea increased by 40 percent. By the fifth day, phagocyte activity had increased 120 percent. When people stopped taking echinacea, immune-cell activity dropped off sharply. After three days, there was no difference in immune-cell activity between the group taking echinacea and the control group.

Leading researchers now feel that echinacea may actually be more of an immune-modulating herb, meaning it has a balancing effect on the immune system. As research continues, this may mean that echinacea may be more valuable than just boosting immune function.

VIRUS SLAYERS

While there are a host of modern antibiotics for killing bacteria, modern medicine has a limited arsenal of weapons to defeat viral infections. This presents a problem for the many doctors who rely on conventional pharmaceuticals in their medical practice. Over 65 million people in the US each year "catch" the common cold, while another 108 million get the flu—and these are just two of the infectious diseases caused by viruses. Others include genital herpes, which affects an estimated 45 million people, as well as hepatitis C, which afflicts 170 million people in the world. Even a simple viral infection like a viral sore throat poses a challenge for any doctor who relies exclusively on antibiotics and other conventional prescription medications.

Echinacea, like some other immune-enhancing herbs, has a direct antiviral effect. Even better, it seems to summon all the resources of the immune system to help destroy viral invaders.

It also works well in combination with other antiviral plants and herbs. I like to prescribe echinacea in a formula called the "virus cocktail," which is comprised of echinacea, lomatium, astragalus, reishi and licorice root. The synergistic blend of these herbs tends to be more effective than any one herb by itself.

BACTERIA AND FUNGUS

Since echinacea enhances the action of your immune cells, it is also effective against bacterial, fungal and yeast infections. This is especially helpful if you're fighting a bacterial infection, because many bacteria are now resistant to antibiotics (because they're overprescribed by doctors for things like viral infections). If needed, there is no problem using echinacea in combination with antibiotics. As a matter of fact, I find when people are on antibiotics for a bacterial infection and use echinacea simultaneously, they recover more quickly.

At least one study—which included 4,190 patients—confirmed this observation. Researchers divided the patients into two groups and gave about half of them an antibacterial formula that included echinacea (along with two other herbs—thuja and baptisia). Along with that formula, the patients received antibiotics that were chosen by the doctors. For comparison, the rest of the patients received only antibiotics, with no herbal formula.

The results showed the effectiveness of taking herbal antibacterial agents along with antibiotics. In the group that got an echinacea-based formula plus an antibiotic, people were cured significantly faster and there was a lower incidence of recurring infection than in the group of people who just got an antibiotic. Also, the symptoms of "sore throat" and "difficulty in swallowing" were improved much more efficiently in the first group than in the second group.

Dosage: Echinacea is generally available as a tincture, capsule, tablet or cream in the U.S. It's also possible to take it in the form of an injection, though this method is mainly used in Germany.

Glycerine (alcohol-free) tinctures are available. These are good for kids, who especially enjoy the berry-flavored varieties.

•**Tincture.** I recommend 20 to 60 drops of the tincture every two to three hours for acute infections or twice daily for long-term use.

•**Capsule.** I recommend 500 to 1,000 milligrams every two to three hours for acute infections or twice daily for long-term use.

Note: High-potency, quality echinacea products are standardized to contain active ingredients such as alkylamides, cichoric acid and polysaccharides.

Some controversy surrounds the length of time one can use echinacea. Many authors state that echinacea should not be used on a long-term basis. However, there are no studies showing that long-term use is harmful or that echinacea loses its effectiveness.

I generally recommend patients use echinacea for acute infections until they are completely over the illness. For those who are very susceptible to infections, especially during the winter, and do not want to change their lifestyle, echinacea can be used on a long-term basis (although it is not so effective as improving diet, reducing stress and exercising). Long-term use of echinacea throughout the winter season is common in European countries.

What are the side effects?: There has been no reported toxicity with echinacea, but two patients of mine have had allergic reactions, with some throat swelling after they started taking echinacea. Such a reaction has the potential of being life-threatening. In both cases, I recommended that my patients avoid using echinacea and switch to other immune-enhancing herbs instead.

Recommendations for...

•**Autoimmune conditions.** There's some controversy about prescribing echinacea to patients who have autoimmune diseases—that is, conditions that become worse when the immune system is overactive. The German Commission E, the government-backed medical board in Germany that helps regulate herbal medicine, recommends that echinacea should not be used in those who have tuberculosis, leukosis, collagenosis, multiple sclerosis, AIDS and HIV, lupus, rheumatoid arthritis and other autoimmune conditions. The assumption is that echinacea will worsen the hypersensitivity of the immune system, causing a flare-up of problems.

While I often agree with many of the Commission E recommendations, many physicians point out that there have not been any studies showing that echinacea is harmful for autoimmune conditions. I have not seen or read any reports where a patient with one of these conditions was made worse from using echinacea, despite the fact that millions of people take it every year.

That said, echinacea would not be my first choice for a condition like multiple sclerosis, rheumatoid arthritis or other autoimmune diseases. But when my patients with these conditions have an acute infection, such as a cold or urinary-tract infection, I do recommend echinacea and other immune-enhancing herbs to fight off the infection. Usually these herbs are helpful; in any case, they don't seem to aggravate the autoimmune disease.

Interestingly, German physicians commonly use echinacea as a topical cream to relieve rheumatoid arthritis symptoms. These same doctors also frequently recommend echinacea be taken internally for its natural anti-inflammatory effects. Furthermore, newer research is showing that many autoimmune conditions are due to the immune system reacting to infectious agents, and cross-reacting with the body's own tissue at the same time. In theory, this would make echinacea helpful for these conditions. More studies are needed to tell us exactly what effect—both good or bad—echinacea has for people with inflammatory or autoimmune conditions.

•**Common cold.** I have found that echinacea can help prevent the common cold as well as reduce the symptoms and shorten the duration—but results differ. Some people respond almost miraculously, while others get no benefits at all. Overall, though, echinacea is more effective than over-the-counter medicines, which only help to reduce some of the symptoms of a cold and do nothing to assist the immune system or battle the infection.

One clinical study looked at the effectiveness of *Echinacea purpurea* for 120 patients who had the initial symptoms of the common cold, with "acute, uncomplicated upper airways infection." When these patients took 20 drops of echinacea every two hours for the first day—and thereafter three times daily—they fared much better than another group that took a placebo. At the end of the 10-day study, patients were questioned about the intensity of their illness and the time it took them to improve. In the echinacea group, people averaged four days to recover, while those in the placebo group took an average of eight days to recover.

•**Flu.** Yes, there are a few antiviral drugs that can help treat the flu. However, the clinical data on these drugs does not impress me very much. The most commonly prescribed drug, amantadine, isn't at all effective in the first two or three days. This is a real drawback because most people experience their worst symptoms during the first 72 hours of a flu attack.

Fortunately, my clinical experience has shown that herbs like echinacea can often help with symptoms the first 24 hours. This is supported by research—but the research also suggests that the size of the dose is an important factor. In a study of 180 men and women between the ages of 18 and 60, researchers compared three different groups. The first group took a placebo. The second got 90 drops of *Echinacea purpurea* every day, which is the equivalent of a 450-milligram dose, while the third group received double that, or 900 milligrams daily. Symptoms of

all participants were evaluated after three to four days and again after eight to ten days. The results showed that 90 drops of tincture had little effect, but the people who took 180 drops were significantly better off, with less-severe symptoms that lasted for a shorter time.

•**Skin conditions.** In North America, echinacea has not quite caught on as a topical treatment for skin conditions. But many European makers of skin products are including the herbal ingredient.

A review of 4,958 clinical cases focused on the effectiveness of echinacea ointment. The main researcher in the study concluded that the ointment was highly effective for many skin conditions. These included 1,453 patients with wounds, 900 with varicose ulcers, 629 with eczema, 26 with burns, 222 with herpes simplex and 212 with inflammatory skin problems. More than 90 percent positive results occurred when the ointment was used to treat burns, wounds and herpes.

•**Vaginitis.** Reoccurring vaginal yeast infections can be quite troublesome for women. One German study looked at 203 women with this condition. Of the 60 women taking echinacea (while the rest took a placebo or other medicines), only 10 had recurrences of yeast infections.

A BOON IN PREGNANCY

Pregnant women have to be careful about anything they eat, which includes supplements, so I'm often asked whether echinacea is safe to use during pregnancy. My answer is yes. Echinacea has a long history of use by herbalists and naturopathic doctors for the treatment of acute infections during pregnancy. If a pregnant woman has a cold, flu or urinary-tract infection, I would not hesitate to recommend echinacea. Side effects or problems with the pregnancy or health of the baby have not been reported. In fact, my wife used echinacea during her entire first pregnancy with no adverse effects.

A study by the Hospital for Sick Children in Toronto, in conjunction with the Canadian Naturopathic College, has confirmed the safety of echinacea use during pregnancy. A group of 206 women who used echinacea during pregnancy for upper-respiratory-tract infections were analyzed along with a control group of 198 pregnant women who had upper-respiratory-tract infections but never used echinacea. The researchers found no association with the use of echinacea and birth defects. There were also no differences in the rate of live births or spontaneous abortions between the two groups.

BENEFITS FOR ATHLETES

Sports medicine specialists studied the effect of echinacea on men who participated in triathlons—those grueling events that involve long-distance swimming, running and cycling. It is well known that triathletes are at an increased risk for infection because they train so exhaustively for each event. Among the participants of the study, some took a placebo, others were given a mineral supplement (43 milligrams of magnesium), while a third group took 8 milliliters of *Echinacea purpurea* daily. All three groups of athletes took the supplements for 28 days before a triathlon.

During training, one-quarter to one-third of the athletes taking a placebo or mineral supplement ended up getting colds. (Those taking magnesium missed 13 days of training, while those in the placebo group missed a total of 24 days.) None of those who were taking echinacea showed any cold symptoms, and none missed any training days.

Ashwagandha—Ancient Remedy for Stress

In the ancient tradition of Ayurvedic medicine—as practiced in India for thousands of years—the herb ashwagandha (*Withania somnifera*) has been used to treat conditions such as fatigue, chronic disease, impotence and waning memory. Now, in the twenty-first-century United States, this well-respected herb has a new and even brighter reputation as a much-needed stress reliever.

Sometimes referred to as *Indian ginseng, winter cherry* or *withania,* ashwagandha herb has many similarities to Chinese ginseng. In Ayurvedic medicine, it may be used to treat a number of other diseases besides those already mentioned—including asthma, bronchitis, psoriasis, arthritis and infertility. Ayurvedic doctors prescribe it in very specific ways that are suited to certain constitutional types. It's often given with the so-called "warming herbs," such as ginger, to increase its tonic effect.

Ashwagandha root differs from Chinese ginseng in having a mild sedative action. This makes it well suited for the Type A person—that is, someone who's always "on the go" at such a high rate that he or she may be headed for burnout.

MULTITONIC

Research shows that this herb is an excellent adaptogen that helps the body cope with physical and mental stress. Studies show that ashwagandha can help people who have exhaustion from chronic stress, weakened immunity (for instance, if they have cancer) and as a tonic for chronic diseases, especially inflammatory disorders.

This herb also has overall benefits for many body systems. Ashwagandha is unique in acting as a tonic to the nervous system, but also has sedative and antiepileptic effects. It mobilizes different components of the immune system to fight invading microbes and has a modulating or balancing effect if you have inflammation.

A number of animal and laboratory studies have shown this herb has antitumor activity. Ashwagandha has also been shown to have antioxidant activity, so it's helpful in protecting brain cells (which could explain why it helps to prevent memory loss). It also stimulates red blood cell production. Ashwagandha is also said to be a rich source of iron, so it's a potential choice for the treatment of iron-deficiency anemia.

Animal studies have shown that it increases thyroid hormone levels.

Over 35 chemical constituents have been isolated in this plant. These include some groups of chemicals such as alkaloids, steroidal lactones, saponins and withanolides.

Ashwagandha has been used in only a few human studies—far outweighed by the number of animal or test-tube studies that have been done. However, it has remained popular and highly valued through thousands of years of use in Ayurvedic medicine. This is a classic case of an herb that has often been used for successful treatments yet never "proven" by modern scientific research. In my opinion, ashwagandha should be used when indicated. I am sure continued scientific research will eventually shed light on the reasons why this wonderful plant has proven so helpful to so many people.

Dosage: The standard adult dosage is 1,000 to 3,000 milligrams daily of the root.

What are the side effects?: No side effects or toxicity have been reported with ashwagandha. Recommendations for…

•**Aging.** For one full year, 3,000 milligrams of purified ashwagandha powder or placebo was given to 101 normal healthy male volunteers, all between the ages of 50 and 59. The herb had some physical effects that slowed the effects of aging for all the men in the study. All men showed significantly increased hemoglobin and red blood cell count. Improvements in nail calcium and cholesterol were also noted. In addition, nearly 72 percent of the men reported improvement in sexual performance.

•**Anemia and slow growth.** Ashwagandha has been shown in two human studies and several animal studies to increase hemoglobin, red blood cell count and serum iron levels. In a scientific trial that continued for 60 days, 58 healthy children between the ages of 8 and 12 were given milk that was treated with fortified ashwagandha (2,000 milligrams a day). The herb improved the health factors that contribute to growth—leading to a significant increase in hemoglobin and albumin. Researchers concluded that ashwagandha can be a growth promoter in children—and they also noted that these children were less likely to have anemia.

•**Arthritis.** Ashwagandha is used in Ayurvedic herbal formulas for the treatment of arthritis and conditions involving inflammation. In a double-blind, placebo-controlled study, 42 people with osteoarthritis were given a formula containing ashwagandha (along with boswellia, turmeric and zinc) for three months. Their health was compared with a control group that received a placebo.

The herbal formula significantly reduced the severity of pain and the degree of disability. There were no significant changes in the control of inflammation, however. For this reason, ashwagandha is mainly used in formulas where inflammation-controlling substances are also part of the mix.

•**Fatigue.** Ashwagandha has been used for the treatment of chronic fatigue, especially in patients who show signs of nervous exhaustion.

•**Memory problems.** Some holistic practitioners recommend ashwagandha for its benefit to the brain. It helps improve the ability to reason and solve problems as well as improve memory. Practitioners of Ayurvedic medicine, who are familiar with these outcomes, often recommend it for patients who are starting to experience memory loss. Studies on rats have shown that it improves cognitive function.

•**Stress.** Ashwagandha appears to help the body cope with the effects of stress more effectively. I am sure that ashwagandha will become as popular as the ginsengs in helping to deal with this all-too-common problem.

Taking a Break Gives New Energy

Timothy B. McCall, MD, an internist, medical editor of *Yoga Journal* and author of *Examining Your Doctors* (Citadel Press) and *Yoga As Medicine* (Bantam). *www. drmccall.com.*

When your body sends you a signal, it's important to listen to it...or it may start talking "louder." Rather than ignoring the signals, consciously choose to take a break. Sometimes you simply need some time to yourself. Cancel that meeting or workout. Instead, curl up on the couch, and settle down with a bowl of steaming soup and a good book. Afterward, if you feel up to it, light your favorite scented candle, put on some quiet music and practice gentle stretches or yoga poses.

AN EASY YOGA MOVE TO RESTORE BALANCE AND ENERGY

According to Timothy B. McCall, MD, former scholar in residence at the Kripalu Center for Yoga and Health in Stockbridge, Massachusetts, yoga can be extremely beneficial when stress or illness threatens to overwhelm us, because it restores and energizes at the same time. In the go-go culture we live in, no matter the obstacle, the inclination is to fight through it...but don't.

Instead, tune in to what you are feeling inside. Listen and respond to your own body.

Most important: Don't overdo.

One of Dr. McCall's favorite restorative yoga positions is "legs-up-the-wall." *He describes the following pose as ideal to calm the nervous system, ease muscle fatigue and restore health...*

•**To begin, find a quiet space** and place a cylindrical yoga bolster or two thick blankets a few inches from a wall.

•**Lie down on the floor,** with your hips elevated on the bolster or blankets, and prop your legs up against the wall so that you are in an "L" position.

•**Adjust your pose (closer to or farther from the wall),** rest your arms above your head or out to the sides and unclench your hands.

•**Once you are completely comfortable, close your eyes and exhale.** Mentally examine your body from head to toe, consciously dissolving the tension throughout. Be aware of your breath as it passes in and out of your body.

•**Rest in this position for as long as you feel comfortable, then slowly open your eyes, straighten up and return to the "real world."** According to Dr. McCall, when you surrender to the softness of this pose, you invite any residual knots of tension to dissolve completely, and it refreshes and renews, empties angst and agitation from the soul, and acts as an antidote to exhaustion, illness and weakened immunity.

Whatever route you decide to take to relaxation and renewal, be it yoga, meditation or a cup of hot tea, make sure that you allow yourself the time to take a break. Sometimes it's all you need to accomplish your goals with even more strength and confidence.

Recommendations for Poor Memory

Do you have a poor memory? *Dr. Stengler recommends the following seven remedies that can help make it better...*

1. Phosphatidylserine. Take 300 milligrams (mg) daily. This naturally occurring phospholipid improves brain cell communication and memory.

2. Bacopa (Bacopa monniera). This nutrient has been shown to improve memory and recall. Take 300 mg daily.

3. Ginkgo biloba (24 percent). Take 120 mg two to three times daily. It improves circulation to the brain, improves memory and has antioxidant benefits.

4. Vitamin B-12. Take 800 to 1600 micrograms (mcg) daily. Consider using a sublingual form at 400 mcg. A vitamin B-12 deficiency contributes to poor memory.

5. Club moss (Huperzia serrata). Take a product standardized to contain 0.2 mg of huperizine A daily. This compound has been shown to increase acetylcholine levels in the brain and to improve memory in people with Alzheimer's disease.

6. Essential fatty acids. Take 1 to 2 tablespoons of flaxseed oil or 2 to 5 grams of fish oil daily. It supplies essential fatty acids for proper brain function.

7. Acetyl-L-carnitine. Take 500 mg three times daily. It improves brain cell communication and memory.

SPECIAL REPORT #3:

New Breakthroughs in Holistic Medicine

New Breakthroughs in Holistic Medicine

Blood Clots and Leg Pain

Carolee, a 61-year-old preschool teacher, had been a patient of mine for the past year. With the help of dietary changes and nutritional supplements, we had made great strides in reducing her weight and controlling her chronic sinusitis and coughing. Unexpectedly, she began experiencing severe pain in her lower right leg during a vacation overseas. Her family took her to a clinic, where blood tests and an ultrasound were performed. The doctor suspected she had *thrombophlebitis* (blood clots in the veins of her legs). Left untreated, this condition can allow clots to travel from the leg and lodge in the blood vessels of the heart or brain, triggering a heart attack or stroke. However, the ultrasound and blood tests came back normal, and Carolee was diagnosed with *phlebitis* (inflammation of the vein) and given *acetaminophen* (Tylenol) for the pain. A week later, she returned to the US and came to my office because she was experiencing a stiff right calf muscle.

Because the results of her ultrasound were normal, I diagnosed Carolee as having chronic venous insufficiency—poor blood flow through the veins of the legs. At the time she had severe pain, there was stress on her circulatory system because she was still somewhat overweight, had taken a long flight (which can impede blood flow), walked more than she usually did and may have been mildly dehydrated. She probably had been suffering a degree of poor circulation for some time, but the symptoms manifested because of the excessive walking she did on her vacation. Poor blood flow could have contributed to the recent stiffness in her calf muscle.

Even though her ultrasound was normal, I was concerned about blood clots. I recommended

Mark A. Stengler, ND, naturopathic physician in private practice, La Jolla, California…adjunct associate clinical professor at the National College of Natural Medicine, Portland, Oregon…author of many books, including *The Natural Physician's Healing Therapies* and coauthor of *Prescription for Natural Cures* (both from Bottom Line Books)…and author of the *Bottom Line/Natural Healing* newsletter.

natto-kinase, a protein-digesting enzyme capsule that improves circulation through blood vessels and breaks down clot-forming proteins. I also asked her to start taking an herbal formula containing horse chestnut extract (made from seeds of the horse chestnut tree)...butcher's broom root extract (a shrub of the lily family)...and gotu kola leaf extract (a perennial plant native to India, China, Australia and parts of South Africa). Horse chestnut and butcher's broom improve the function of vein valves, so that they prevent the backflow of venous blood. Gotu kola strengthens vein walls, so that they don't distend and pool blood. Carolee had access to a whirlpool tub, so I recommended that four times each day she alternate sitting on the side with her legs in the whirlpool for two minutes and putting her legs in the nearby pool's cooler water for 30 seconds. Alternating hot and cold and the massaging action of the whirlpool improves circulation. Exercise and elevation are recommended for people who don't have access to whirlpools.

Carolee reported great improvement within one week and had no remaining symptoms one month later. She continues to take the supplements to prevent the problem from recurring.

Natural Help for Incontinence

With a grimace, Peter, 79, tugged at his waistband and growled, "It's darned inconvenient running to the bathroom every half hour during the day and four times each night. And I hate wearing this so-called 'absorbent undergarment.' I feel like a baby wetting his diapers!"

Peter's urinary incontinence had begun three years earlier, after a cancer diagnosis and surgery to remove his prostate gland. He also had Parkinson's disease (a neurological disorder that impairs movement control). Medications helped to ease some of his Parkinson's symptoms, but the disease exacerbated his incontinence.

Temporary or chronic urinary incontinence affects one in five adults over age 40, primarily women. It can result from pelvic injury or surgery...pregnancy, childbirth or menopause... and/or neurological diseases, infection or aging.

For Peter, I prescribed a liquid formula of extracts from six safe herbs that I have used with a number of my patients—male and female—over the past several years. It is called Bladder Tonic by Wise Woman Herbals (800-277-9861, *www.houseofnutrition.com*). These herbs have a long history of successful use by naturopathic doctors and herbalists.

• **Lady's mantle** is believed to strengthen the muscles of the bladder (so it is better able to hold urine) and of the sphincter that controls the *urethra* (the tube that drains urine out of the body).

• **Partridge berry** also may improve the bladder's muscular tone.

• **Gotu kola** (a perennial plant native to Asia) may strengthen the bladder's connective tissue.

• **St. John's wort** (known for its antidepressant effect) may soothe irritated nerves of the urinary tract. (It should not be used by people who take antidepressant drugs or birth control pills.)

• **Witch hazel** eases inflammation and tightens lax (loose) tissues of the bladder.

• **Corn silk** soothes tissues and reduces urinary tract inflammation.

Formulas similar to the one I prescribe for my incontinent patients are sold at health-food stores or through herbalists and naturopathic physicians.

Recommended: One teaspoonful twice daily, mixed with water. Other than very occasional and mild stomach upset from the corn silk, side effects are rare, and these herbs are safe for everyone (except pregnant and nursing women, who should avoid them as a general precaution).

After six weeks on this regimen, Peter returned for a follow-up visit feeling extremely encouraged. He was urinating only half as often during the day, so he could pursue his activities with fewer interruptions, and his nighttime need for the toilet was somewhat improved. Although he still wore a protective undergarment as a precaution, Peter was satisfied. "No more wet baby," he laughed. "I feel like a man again."

Omega-3 Fatty-Acid Levels May Be Low in Vegetarians

By now, you have probably heard that omega-3 fatty acids in the diet can help prevent several chronic conditions, such as cardiovascular disease, osteoporosis and certain cancers, in particular breast, colon and prostate malignancies.

Fish such as wild salmon, sardines, trout, tuna, herring, mackerel and shellfish and supplemental fish oil capsules are by far the richest sources of the omega-3 fatty acids known as DHA (*docosahexaenoic acid*) and EPA (*eicosapentaenoic acid*).

So what can vegans (people who strictly avoid all animal products, including dairy, eggs and fish in their diet) and vegetarians (those who avoid meat and poultry but eat dairy, eggs and fish) do to obtain enough of these healthful fatty acids? Reports suggest that vegans and vegetarians have significantly lower levels of omega-3s in their blood than meat eaters. In a recent study, researchers at Oxford University and King's College, both in England, compared the plasma fatty-acid composition in 196 meat eaters, 231 vegetarians and 232 vegan men in the UK. They found that when meat is entirely excluded from the diet, the body has lower concentrations of DHA and EPA.

Therefore, one of my concerns about vegan and vegetarian diets is the potential for a deficiency of DHA and EPA. These "good fats" are very important for key organs, such as the heart (to prevent stroke and reduce inflammation of blood vessels)…eyes (for the formation of eye receptors)…brain (to help with memory and focus)…bones (to prevent osteoporosis)…and joints (to lubricate and reduce inflammation of the joints).

I suggest that vegans and vegetarians supplement with flaxseed oil or hemp oil—one tablespoon of either daily. The body can convert the omega-3s in these plant oils into DHA and EPA.

Nature's Virus Killers for Colds and Flu

Do you have to get a cold or the flu this coming season? No! This year can be different. With the right preparation, quick intervention and a lineup of powerful, natural virus fighters, there's a good chance that you can enjoy fall and winter without getting sick. *Here's how…*

KNOW YOUR ENEMY

Colds and flu are both caused by viruses. They are spread through the air by coughs and sneezes and through contact with contaminated objects, such as a doorknob or a hand that has been used to cover a cough. A virus is little more than a clump of genetic material (DNA or RNA) inside a packet made of protein. Stray viruses constantly land on your body. The trouble starts when they attach to cell receptors and get inside your cells. Viruses use the cells' own reproductive equipment to duplicate themselves—damaging more and more cells as they churn out millions of lookalikes.

It actually is a good sign when you begin to get a stuffy head or a runny nose. Your body is fighting back. Your immune system picks up signals from the by-products of viral activity—pain, redness, swelling, heat, fever and rash are results of your immune system launching a counterattack. Mucus is produced to help expel viral intruders.

Flu viruses are a lot more powerful than typical cold viruses. Cold symptoms are mainly confined to the head, neck and chest. Flu causes more generalized symptoms, such as fever, body aches, nausea, cramping, vomiting and severe fatigue. Flu also can develop into bronchitis. In the worst cases, it can lead to pneumonia and other severe respiratory diseases that are sometimes fatal, especially in the elderly or others with weakened immune systems.

New threat: Avian flu has been a problem in Asia and has the potential to reach the US. Because it also is caused by a virus, I would recommend the same natural approach that can be used for the regular flu.

START WITH PREVENTION

I'll tell you about great ways to feel better if you get a cold or flu, but prevention should be your first line of defense…

 •**Avoid spending time around people who already are sick,** particularly if they're coughing or sneezing. If you live with someone who is sick, sleep in separate rooms. Wash your hands frequently during cold-and-flu season, and don't share towels—assign one to each family member or use paper towels. Keep your hands away from your face, especially your nose, mouth and eyes.

 •**Take vitamins.** A good multivitamin/mineral supplement provides a base of nutrients to support a healthy immune system. A formula that I recommend as a preventive against viral infections is Source Naturals Wellness Formula (to find a retailer near you, call 800-815-2333 or go to *www.sourcenaturals.com*). It contains vitamins A and C, which are involved in the formation of antibodies…the minerals zinc and selenium… and immune-supportive herbs, such as garlic, echinacea and astragalus, which increase the activity of virus-fighting white blood cells. The dosage used to prevent infection is two capsules daily during cold-and-flu season, taken in conjunction with your year-round multisupplement.

 •**Reduce exposure to toxins.** You are more vulnerable to viral infection when your body is "distracted" by having to deal with toxins that can damage or suppress the immune system. Toxins aren't necessarily exotic—they could include sugars and alcohol consumed to excess, fast food and other unhealthy food laced with artificial preservatives and/or pesticides. Smoking and second-hand smoke injures the respiratory tract and makes you and your children more susceptible to colds and flus. Toxins also include small but significant amounts of metals—mercury, arsenic and lead—that you can get from food, water and air pollution.

It is even more vital to eat healthfully during cold-and-flu season because you're indoors more and are exposed to higher concentrations of germs. Go easy on holiday sweets and other treats, and you will be less likely to get sick.

Many people cut back their exercise regimens in winter months—a big mistake, since exercise strengthens your immune system. Also consider sitting in a dry sauna once or twice a week for 20 to 30 minutes…or a wet sauna for 10 to 15 minutes. Saunas increase sweating, which excretes toxins. Be sure to check with your doctor first if you have diabetes or heart disease.

For those who get colds or the flu every year, I recommend taking a super-greens formula in the fall to remove toxins from the colon, liver and lymphatic system. It also can be taken year-round for gentle continuous detoxification. One good product is Greens+ (800-643-1210, *www.greensplus.com*), which contains chlorella, wheat grass, super-green foods and detoxifying herbs such as milk thistle. The dosage is one scoop a day dissolved in water or juice.

Don't forget the impact that toxic emotions have on your immune system. Anger, anxiety, resentment, loneliness and other chronic emotional difficulties trigger the release of hormones that suppress immune function. Seek support to overcome these problems if they linger.

DO CONVENTIONAL THERAPIES HELP?

At the first sign of a runny nose or scratchy throat, some people head straight to the drugstore for cold and flu remedies. However, there are no conventional drugs—available either by prescription or over the counter—that help cure the common cold. Nasal decongestants and pain medications may make you feel better, but they don't address the actual viral infection. Natural remedies also can help you feel better—with fewer potential side effects—and they simultaneously improve immune function.

For flu, on the other hand, a number of effective prescription antiviral drugs are available that may reduce the flu's severity and duration (by one or two days) if taken within 48 hours of the first signs of illness. Such medicines include *amantadine* (Symmetrel), *rimantadine* (Flumadine), *zanamivir* (Relenza) and *oseltamivir* (Tamiflu). Possible short-term side effects range from central nervous system problems, including anxiety and light-headedness, to decreased respiratory function and digestive upset. These antiviral drugs are not approved for children under age one.

All of these antiviral drugs except zanamivir also are approved for *preventing* the flu during outbreaks. These may benefit individuals who are immunocompromised—for example, those who have AIDS or have had organ or bone transplants. I prefer to have my otherwise healthy patients focus on effective natural therapies since they work so well and rarely cause side effects.

RELY ON NATURE'S VIRUS KILLERS

If you start to come down with a cold or the flu, my first recommendation is to change your diet. Eat lightly so that your body can focus on healing. For the first 24 hours, consume filtered water, broths and soups with lots of garlic, onions and spices, such as turmeric and cayenne, which relieve congestion, promote circulation and have a natural anti-inflammatory effect. Herbal teas (especially ginger, cinnamon and peppermint) and steamed vegetables also are good choices. When you're feeling better, move toward a more normal diet.

I have found several supplements to be effective for treating colds and flu. Consider taking these when people around you are sick or when you first feel cold and flu symptoms that can include fever (flu), headache (flu), fatigue, stuffy nose, sneezing, sore throat, chest discomfort, coughing and general aches and pains. You can use one or any combination until you feel better.

•**Lomatium dissectum** is a plant once used by Native Americans to fight Spanish flu. Preliminary research shows that lomatium has the ability to prevent viruses from replicating and to stimulate white blood cell activity. With colds and flu, I often see improvement within 24 hours. In my experience, the only side effect has been an allergic reaction in the form of a measleslike rash in a small percentage of users. This rash disappears a few days after lomatium is discontinued.

Eclectic Institute makes a potent product called Lomatium-Osha (800-332-4372, *www.eclecticherb. com*), which soothes the respiratory tract. This product is 50% alcohol, so take only the dosage recommended on the label. Women who are pregnant or nursing should not use lomatium.

•**Elderberry,** as shown by research in Israel, can stimulate the immune system, enhance white blood cell activity and inhibit viral replication. Flu patients have reported significant improvement within 48 hours of taking elderberry. It also helps with colds. The elderberry used in research studies is Sambucol Black Elderberry Extract from Nature's Way (to find a retailer, call

800-962-8873 or go to *www.naturesway.com*). Adults should take two teaspoons four times daily…children, one teaspoon four times daily.

•**Echinacea,** contrary to recent media reports, can be effective for treating colds and flu. Echinacea makes the body's own immune cells more efficient in attacking viruses. The key is using a product that has been processed to contain a high level of active constituents. Ground-up echinacea root or leaves won't do much. The use of alcohol and water by the manufacturer to extract active components is critical to the product's potency. Also, be sure to use enough (many people don't). Two potent, well-researched products are Echinamide: Fresh Alcohol-Free Echinacea Extract, Natural Berry Flavor, and Echinamide Anti-V Formula Softgels, both by Natural Factors (to find a retailer, call 800-322-8704 or go to *www.naturalfactors.com*). This echinacea has been shown to reduce the length and severity of the common cold.

If you feel a cold or the flu coming on, take 20 drops of liquid extract or two capsules every two waking hours for 24 hours, then cut back to every three waking hours until the illness has passed.

The same company makes a liquid preparation called Anti-V Formula, which contains Echinamide, lomatium and other virus fighters. It is the most aggressive product for cold and flu from the Natural Factors line and can be used instead of the other supplements. Take 1.5 ml every two waking hours for the first 48 hours and then every three waking hours until the illness is gone.

•**Homeopathic influenzinum** is an intriguing remedy that I have used with success. Made from active flu strains, it stimulates the body's own defense system to resist infection. It works along the same lines as an oral vaccine, but since it is homeopathic, none of the flu particles are left in the preparation. It can be used for prevention or treatment of flu and has no side effects.

Take two 30C-potency pellets twice daily for two weeks at the beginning of flu season (in early November). Take two pellets four times daily when exposed to flu sufferers or if you start to have symptoms. It is available from health-food stores and The Vitamin Shoppe (866-293-3367, *www.vitaminshoppe.com*).

•**Oscillococcinum** is another great homeopathic remedy for flu, which is also available from The Vitamin Shoppe, health-food stores and pharmacies or by calling 800-672-4556 or visiting *www.oscillo.com.* It can be taken at the first sign of flu and is the number-one–selling homeopathic flu remedy in the US.

•**N-acetylcysteine (NAC)** helps thin the mucus that may accompany a cold or the flu. In addition to making you feel better, NAC helps to prevent sinus and more serious chest infections. A study at University of Genoa, Italy, showed that NAC, when taken as a supplement, could help prevent as well as treat flu. The nutrient increases levels of the powerful antioxidant *glutathione* in the body, which, in turn, improves immune function. NAC is available at any health-food store and many pharmacies. If you tend to get the flu every year, take 600 mg twice daily when you are around people who have the flu or if you start feeling sick yourself.

•**Vitamin C** enhances the activity of white blood cells. I have found that taking 3,000 mg to 5,000 mg daily helps fight viral infections. However, some people get diarrhea from this amount. For immediate treatment of symptoms, start with 5,000 mg in divided doses. If loose stools occur, cut back to 3,000 mg (or even less).

Fixing Fatigue After a Quadruple Bypass

Many who've been through bypass surgery experience uncomfortable after-effects like shortness of breath and fatigue. Some patients have reported that taking hawthorn improves these symptoms, but there are other supplements to be considered as well.

Coenzyme Q10 (300 mg daily) and *L-carnitine* (2,000 mg) are nutrients that help the heart contract with better force. Studies have shown that they can improve congestive heart failure. Another supplement I strongly recommend is ribose at a dosage of 5 g taken twice daily. This nutrient helps heart cells produce energy more effectively. A European study found that ribose

supplementation significantly improved heart function in cardiac patients.

Magnesium also is critical to proper heart function. A good dosage is 250 mg to 400 mg twice daily. In addition, I have written about the mushroom cordyceps in the past and how it supports heart function. The recommended dosage is 1,500 mg to 1,600 mg twice daily of the Cs-4 extract. Be sure to talk with your cardiologist before taking any supplements. You also may want to consult with your cardiologist about enhanced external counterpulsation (EECP). This involves the use of pressure cuffs on the legs that are inflated by a machine in sequences. The blood vessels in the legs are gently compressed, which improves the rate at which blood returns to the heart.

"Full-Body" CT Scans

It wasn't so long ago that a Cat scan—a computerized X-ray technique, also called a CT (for "computed tomography") scan—seemed very exotic. In fact, if you're age 35 or older, there were no CT scanners in clinical use when you were born. Today, of course, CT scans are commonplace.

Now there's an even more advanced, and highly touted, version—electron beam computed tomography (EBCT), often (erroneously) referred to as a full-body scan. EBCT scans examine the abdominal cavity and chest (including coronary arteries and lungs). These scans are available in cities nationwide and are being promoted as a way to detect coronary artery disease and other abnormalities, including tumors and aneurysms in the chest, abdomen and pelvic area. In many states, a prescription is not required to get a scan. Even if you're healthy, you can just contact an imaging center and ask—and pay—for the test. The idea is to find trouble before any symptoms appear.

EBCT scans use very rapidly processed X-rays that capture images in a fraction of a second. This allows for clear, freeze-frame pictures of the heart and arteries while the heart is beating. Images are captured from many angles, allowing a three-dimensional view of the heart as well as other organs and systems.

The test is painless. While the patient lies on a table, an overhead scan machine takes images in an open environment—not in an enclosed space as with some other CT and magnetic resonance imaging (MRI) scans. Testing usually takes 10 to 15 minutes. Typically, a center's radiologist or cardiologist determines if there are any visible abnormalities and reviews the results with the patient within minutes. Upon your request, a copy of the report and images can be sent to your primary care doctor.

One purpose of an EBCT scan is to determine the amount of calcium buildup in the lining of the arteries, including the coronary arteries. Several studies, including one conducted at the respected Cooper Institute in Dallas and published last year in the *American Journal of Epidemiology*, have shown a correlation between the degree of calcification and the severity of hardening of the arteries, known as atherosclerosis. A low level of calcium buildup in the arteries means that your risk for coronary artery disease is low. A high level means that you are at higher risk for cardiovascular problems in the future.

There are a few downsides to EBCT scans. One is the radiation exposure from the X-rays—which can be two to 10 times more than that of a standard X-ray. Radiation is a known risk factor for cancer (although the risk appears small with occasional scans). The EBCT scan also may result in "false positives"—meaning that doctors may spot a suspected lesion that requires follow-up tests, possibly even an invasive biopsy and it may turn out to be nothing serious. Lastly, many insurance companies don't cover EBCT preventive screening. A scan costs $850 to $1,500.

Despite the financial cost, I do recommend that people age 40 and older get a preventive EBCT screening. If the results are normal, then follow up with another in five to 10 years. The test is even more important for those with a strong family history of heart disease or cancer. While EBCT scanning is not foolproof, it can help detect life-threatening diseases that are best treated with early intervention.

Ginkgo Biloba— A Power Plant

While ginkgo may well be the most widely publicized herb to come along in the past 50 years, the history of its healing powers certainly predates its current popularity. In fact, the Chinese have known about it and have used it for over 3,500 years.

Ginkgo ranks among the top five herbs that I prescribe to patients on a daily basis. Millions of people around the world use ginkgo every day. In countries such as Germany and France, where doctors are accustomed to writing herbal prescriptions, ginkgo is among the most commonly prescribed medicines. European doctors use it to treat a wide range of conditions—from memory impairment, dizziness and ringing in the ears (tinnitus) to headaches and depression. There are even more uses—such as a blood mover for improved circulation.

If ginkgo trees could speak for themselves, some would give first-person accounts of Aztecs, Vikings and the Battle of Hastings, since the grandparents of the species have lived as long as 1,000 years. Some reach a height of 120 feet, with a girth of 48 inches. Apart from longevity, ginkgoes boast venerable ancestors.

Fossil records show that the ginkgo is the world's oldest living species of tree. It's very hardy, able to thrive in extreme heat and cold, and to withstand the sinus-hammering pollution of downtown Los Angeles or New York. It's also almost pest-proof—there doesn't seem to be an insect that can do serious damage to this hardy tree.

The leaves, the source of ginkgo medicinals, are fan-shaped and bilobed, resembling the maidenhair fern. The resemblance is so close, it's sometimes called the "maidenhair tree."

TURNING OVER AN OLD LEAF...

Researchers in the 1950s, having heard of the medicinal powers of ginkgo (tree) leaves, began mashing and distilling the components in search of the so-called active ingredients—that is, the chemical compounds that seemed to have potential healing power. What are believed to be the key medicinal ingredients have now been identified. I know it would be rash to say these are all the active, healing constituents—certainly more will be discovered—but at least we're starting to understand how some of the ginkgo-leaf ingredients make important contributions to improved health.

While the active constituents are important, however, I remind people that it's best to use the whole herb rather than focus on one ingredient or component. Studies have shown, however, that the whole herb plus standardized active constituents are more effective than just using the isolated active constituents.

The two groups of active components include flavone glycosides and terpene lactones. Quality ginkgo products are "standardized" to 24% flavone glycosides and 6% terpene lactones—which is a virtual guarantee that the products contain at least these proportions of those particular ingredients. Such products have the same proportion of these ingredients as the extract that's used in clinical studies.

POTENT CELL PROTECTOR...

Flavone glycosides are types of *bioflavonoids,* the plant-based compounds that are found in oranges and other fruits and vegetables. With bioflavonoids, ginkgo has been blessed with the potent powers of an antioxidant. That means if you take ginkgo, you're less likely to suffer the cellular damage caused by free radicals—unstable molecules that are a result of metabolic activities in the body and environmental pollution.

Many researchers believe that ginkgo produces more antioxidant activity than many of the better-known vitamin antioxidants such as C, E and beta carotene. Several studies have demonstrated that ginkgo exerts antioxidant activity in the brain, eyes and cardiovascular system. This could easily explain why ginkgo seems to be effective in the prevention and treatment of diseases that affect those parts of the body—including Alzheimer's disease, strokes, cataracts, macular degeneration and diabetic retinopathy.

Ginkgo bioflavonoids also protect blood vessels by strengthening and reducing inflammation of their elastic walls. So that's an additional benefit of this herb—significant in helping to relieve varicose veins and reverse the effects of cardiovascular disease.

KEEPING UP CIRCULATION...

In addition to the bioflavonoids, ginkgo has another component, unique to this plant. A family of terpene lactones, specifically called *ginkgolides* and *bilobalides,* give ginkgo an extraordinary ability to increase circulation to the brain and extremities. The substances cause the blood vessel walls to relax and dilate, which permits increased blood flow. They also have what's called a "tonifying effect" on the venous system, allowing for the more efficient return of blood to the heart.

Ginkgo also has a natural blood-thinning effect. It helps to prevent blood platelets from sticking together—and platelets are the cells that form blood clots.

The way ginkgo improves circulation is particularly impressive. In one study where researchers measured the blood flow through capillaries in healthy adults, they found a 57 percent increase in blood flow among those who were regularly taking ginkgo. This finding is particularly important to seniors. As we age, we're more likely to have blockages in the blood flow that reaches the brain and other parts of the bodies. These problems are directly attributable to plaque buildup in the arteries. Ginkgo acts as sort of a bypass mechanism, helping the blood make its way through partially clogged arteries.

NERVE RENEWAL...

The ginkgolides also help protect nerve cells from being damaged. This is important for people who are recovering from a stroke. In addition, some ongoing research will probably show whether ginkgo has the benefits that it's reputed to possess for people who are recovering from brain trauma. What's certain is that nerve cells need the kind of protection that ginkgo provides—particularly people (such as those with diabetes) who have problems with neuropathy (nerve disorder).

Dosage: As a standard dosage, I recommend a ginkgo extract standardized to 24% flavone glycosides and 6% terpene lactones. Dosages used in studies range from 120 milligrams to 360 milligrams daily. Most of my patients take 60 milligrams two to four times daily, for a daily total of 120 to 240 milligrams. The vast majority report beneficial results.

For severe cases, like early-stage Alzheimer's disease, I recommend that people take 240 to 360 milligrams daily.

If you start to take ginkgo for a particular condition or for general health, I suggest you continue taking it for at least eight weeks to assess its therapeutic effect. Most of my patients who take it to improve their memory or help their circulation notice the beginnings of improvements within about a month.

Ginkgo supplements are available in capsule, tablet and tincture form.

What are the side effects: Doctors, researchers and practitioners have noted very few adverse effects among people who take ginkgo. A small number—less than 1 percent of those who take it—have reported mild digestive upset.

Other rare side effects mentioned in the literature include headaches and dizziness. I've had very few patients who complained of these problems, and in those few cases, the side effects disappeared when I lowered the dosage.

One warning, however. If you're taking a blood-thinning medication such as Coumadin or aspirin, be sure to notify your doctor. These medications, like ginkgo, have a blood-thinning effect—and the cumulative doses might be more than you need. Your doctor can monitor how well your blood is clotting through regular blood work, by taking blood samples and testing them in the lab.

Recommendations for…

•Attention Deficit Disorder (ADD). Although I have not seen any studies on ginkgo and Attention Deficit Disorder, I have had parents tell me that it helps their children with concentration and memory with schoolwork. These are specifically children with memory and concentration problems—not hyperactivity.

•Alzheimer's disease. Ginkgo has shown to be of benefit in cases of senility and Alzheimer's disease. In fact, it has been approved for the treatment of Alzheimer's disease by the German government. While it's not a cure—none exists—ginkgo has been shown effective in delaying the mental deterioration that often occurs rapidly in the early stage of the disease.

A study done in 1994, involving 40 patients who had early-stage Alzheimer's disease, demonstrated that 240 milligrams of ginkgo biloba extract taken daily for 3 months produced measurable improvements in memory, attention and mood.

Most of the patients I see do not have Alzheimer's, but they experience a general decline in short-term memory and concentration. Ginkgo is at the top of the list for safe and effective supplements I recommend. Plus, it is not overly expensive—about $12 to $16 per month at the dosage I recommend—so you won't break the bank if you take it regularly.

•Circulatory diseases. Ginkgo is one of the best medicines in the world for improving circulation to the hands and feet. For this reason it's an effective treatment for intermittent claudication.

People who have intermittent claudication—which is really a circulatory problem—experience pain and severe cramping in the lower legs, particularly while walking. This condition is particularly prevalent among the elderly. Many clinical studies have shown ginkgo can help alleviate the condition in 3 to 6 months if you take daily dosages of 120 to 160 milligrams.

Ginkgo has also been shown to improve the condition of people who have Raynaud's disease, a condition where the hands or feet instantly turn blue if you just reach for something in the freezer or step outside on a cold day. (For some reason, women are much more likely than men to suffer from this condition.) Again, the problem is circulatory. I have frequently recommended ginkgo—and achieved positive results—when patients were bothered by cold hands and feet.

Finally, people with diabetes are particularly prone to have poor circulation in their extremities. Supplementing with ginkgo is certainly beneficial.

•Depression. Ginkgo is an effective natural antidepressant when the depression is related to poor blood flow to the brain. When blood flow improves, more oxygen and nutrients naturally reach the brain cells as well as extremities.

Ginkgo also improves the activity of neurotransmitters, the brain's chemical messengers. A study of elderly patients who took doses of 240 milligrams of ginkgo extract daily showed that many experienced significant improvements in mood after only 4 weeks. The improvements were even more dramatic after 8 weeks of taking the same concentration of extract.

•**High blood pressure.** Ginkgo is one of the main herbs I recommend to patients who have hypertension or high blood pressure. It helps to relax the artery walls, thus reducing pressure within the blood vessels. A typical dosage would be 120 to 180 milligrams daily.

•**Impotence.** Impotence occurs in the vast majority of cases because there's poor circulation to erectile tissue. Instead of recommending Viagra to patients with impotence problems, I usually start with a prescription of ginkgo biloba (and sometimes some ginseng as well). Ginkgo works very well, is much less expensive, and doesn't have any side effects—unlike Viagra.

Because ginkgo improves penile blood flow, it provides the physiological basis for an erection. In one study, 50 percent of patients treated for impotence using 60 milligrams of ginkgo per day regained potency.

I generally recommend 180 to 240 milligrams of ginkgo in the treatment of impotence. If ginkgo doesn't help, I'll have the patient tested for the hormones DHEA and testosterone. If these hormones are deficient, I'll recommend they be used in therapeutic dosages.

•**Memory loss.** Even if you don't remember things so well as you used to, the awareness of memory loss is not a signal of oncoming Alzheimer's disease or senility. Memory loss is quite common—and understandable, given the fact that we do tend to lose some memory capacity as we age and that we are quite susceptible to distractions.

"Cerebral vascular insufficiency" is a phrase that's often used to describe poor blood flow to the brain. Often, the problem gets worse as people get older because people gradually experience atherosclerosis—hardening of the arteries—which sharply decreases the efficiency of blood flow. Simply put, when the brain doesn't get enough oxygenated, nourishing blood, we're more likely to have memory loss. (Depression, as noted, can also be related to restricted blood flow.) Given its power to improve blood flow, ginkgo biloba is the treatment of choice. Once the brain cells get the oxygen and blood sugar needed to help them function properly, memory improves. Clinical studies have confirmed that

significant change can occur as rapidly as 8 to 12 weeks.

•**Premenstrual syndrome (PMS).** For women who experience cramping, pain and breast tenderness around the time of their periods, ginkgo may also provide some benefits. I have been surprised to learn that these typical symptoms of PMS might respond to ginkgo. Studies have shown that ginkgo can be helpful in alleviating breast tenderness and fluid retention.

•**Radiation effects.** After the Chernobyl nuclear accident in 1986, Russian scientists tried a wide variety of treatments to help workers and residents who had been exposed to radiation. Researchers discovered that ginkgo helped combat the effects of radiation. It was found to be a potent agent in fighting free-radical damage to the cells, providing the same antioxidant benefits that help protect normal body cells from the effects of rapid aging.

•**Ringing in the ears (tinnitus).** Studies have been done to test the effectiveness of ginkgo in relieving the condition known as tinnitus, which is ringing in the ears. Results have been mixed. I feel it is worth trying if there's the possibility that tinnitus is the result of poor circulation. Sometimes the condition is related to the fact that insufficient blood is reaching the inner ear. In other cases, however, tinnitus occurs when people are exposed to excessive noise—and in those cases, ginkgo doesn't seem to help very much.

Ginkgo can be helpful if you've had acute hearing loss as a result of pressure changes or sound trauma. Even if you don't know the factors that have contributed to loss of hearing, taking this herb might produce some positive effects.

•**Stroke.** Ginkgo is valuable both in the immediate treatment of stroke and in helping stroke victims during the months or years of recovery. One of the keys to the prevention of stroke is keeping the blood thin. Again, the objective is to improve circulation so sufficient blood gets to the brain. New research is also showing that therapeutic doses of antioxidants may be an important treatment for strokes. As I mentioned, ginkgo provides antioxidant activity as well.

Many doctors who are oriented toward holistic medicine—treatment of the whole patient rather than a single "problem"—often recommend ginkgo to people who are particularly susceptible to a stroke. Among those who need to take special care are anyone with a personal or family history of high blood pressure, atherosclerosis, diabetes—particularly if you're a smoker or if you've had a previous stroke. But remember, many doctors prescribe pharmaceutical blood-thinning medications after a stroke, so if you're taking one of these, you need to talk to your doctor and have some blood work done before you start taking ginkgo, too.

•**Vision.** Ginkgo is also useful in the prevention and treatment of macular degeneration and diabetic retinopathy. If left untreated, both conditions can result in blindness. Macular degeneration, often associated with age, is the result of nerve degeneration in the particularly sensitive light-receptor cells of the eye. Diabetic retinopathy is a serious eye disease that can lead to blindness.

Ginkgo has been shown to be helpful in both conditions. I also recommend ginkgo as part of a natural treatment for cataracts.

Plundering the Pineapple For Bromelain

Bromelain is actually a group of protein enzymes derived from the pineapple plant, whose healing powers were described in medical literature as far back as 1876. Though the active enzymes are found in the fruit as well as the stem, commercial products are made exclusively from the stem.

Bromelain is used for many purposes—as a digestive aid, natural blood thinner, anti-inflammatory, mucus-thinning agent, immune-system enhancer and for skin healing. It also helps improve the absorption of certain supplements (such as glucosamine) and drug medications such as antibiotics.

One of bromelain's unique actions is to reduce inflammation in people who have conditions such as arthritis or heart disease. It can also help control the inflammatory process after an injury. It breaks down blood clots at the site of an injury, so swelling is reduced and, at the same time, there's increased circulation to the site of injury or inflammation. Bromelain also helps control some of the body's naturally produced chemicals that tend to increase an inflammatory reaction after an injury.

MAXING YOUR ANTIBIOTICS...

Bromelain is used in many countries to increase the absorption and utilization of antibiotics.

In one study, 53 hospitalized patients were given bromelain in various combinations with appropriate antibiotic medications. Their conditions included a wide range of health problems, including pneumonia, bronchitis, skin staphylococcus infection, thrombophlebitis, cellulitis, pyelonephritis (kidney infection) and abscesses of the rectum. Twenty-three of the patients had been on antibiotic therapy without success. Bromelain was administered four times a day along with antibiotics or by itself.

To compare, a control group of 56 patients was treated with antibiotics alone.

Of the 23 patients who had been unsuccessfully treated with antibiotics, 22 responded favorably to the combined treatment. The rate of improvement was across-the-board, for every type of disease, when patients were given the combination of bromelain and antibiotics.

For doctors involved in the study, it was an eye-opener. Many had not realized that bromelain was able to potentiate the effects of antibiotics in this way.

I hope we'll see larger-scale studies in the near future. Such promising results suggest that people may be able to take lower doses of antibiotics if they simultaneously take bromelain. (Many doctors are eager to reduce the rampant overuse of antibiotics, which is leading to ominous new strains of resistant bacteria.)

Those with weak or compromised immune systems could be the greatest beneficiaries of combination treatments with bromelain and antibiotics. Infants, seniors and AIDS patients are particularly good candidates for the combined therapies.

Dosage: The dosage of bromelain is designated in two different ways with regard to supplements. One is milk-clotting units (M.C.U.) and the other is gelatin-dissolving units (G.D.U.). Look for products that are standardized to 2,000 M.C.U. per 1,000 mg, or 1,200 G.D.U. per 1,000 mg. Most people require a dosage of 500 mg three times daily between meals.

What are the side effects?: Side effects are rare with bromelain. However, allergic reactions can occur in sensitive individuals. Increased heart rate and palpitations have been observed in some people at dosages near 2,000 mg. Those on blood-thinning medications should check with their doctor first before using bromelain.

Recommendations for…

•Arthritis. Bromelain is a popular component of natural arthritis formulas. It is helpful for both osteoarthritis and rheumatoid arthritis.

One study found that the supplementation of bromelain enabled people with rheumatoid arthritis to reduce their corticosteroid medications. In addition, patients noticed significant improvements in joint mobility and also noticed less swelling. This study is encouraging because many people suffer side effects from corticosteroid therapy—and the less medicine they have to use, the better. If bromelain supplementation can reduce the amount of steroids needed, the risk of serious side effects decreases as well.

My experience is that most people with arthritis can maintain a good quality of life if they take the opportunity to try bromelain and other natural treatments.

•Burns. A specially prepared bromelain cream has been shown to eliminate burn debris and speed up the healing of burned skin.

•Cancer. Various studies have looked at a link between bromelain treatments and cancer deterrence or recovery. In one study, 12 patients with ovarian and breast tumors were given 600 mg of bromelain daily for at least 6 months. (Some treatments continued for several years.) Resolution of cancerous masses and a decrease in metastasis was reported.

Bromelain in doses of over 1,000 mg daily have been given in combination with chemotherapy drugs such as 5-FU and vincristine, with some reports of tumor regression.

Although I do not rate bromelain as one of the more potent anti-cancer herbs, it is worthy of more study. For those who are using chemotherapy to fight cancer, the addition of bromelain offers the promise of making the therapy more effective.

•Cardiovascular disease. Holistic practitioners have expressed a great deal of interest in using bromelain for treatment and prevention of cardiovascular disease. We know that bromelain helps break down fibrinous plaques in the arteries, allowing for more efficient circulation. In theory, at least, this is a sure way to help prevent strokes.

When we take routine tests to determine whether people are at risk of cardiovascular disease, fibrin is one of the markers that we're beginning to look at routinely. (In other words, a lot of fibrin in the blood is one indicator that stroke could be somewhere on the horizon.) The fact that bromelain can help "break down" this fibrin is significant. In one study, bromelain administered at a dosage of 400 to 1,000 mg per day to 14 patients with angina (chest pain) resulted in the disappearance of symptoms in all patients within 4 to 90 days.

Bromelain also has the potential to break down plaque, the fatty deposits that impair blood flow through the arteries. The enzyme has been shown to dissolve arteriosclerotic plaque in rabbit heart arteries. While more studies need to be done, I've talked to many practitioners who notice that their patients with heart problems do better on bromelain.

•Digestive problems. Bromelain has long been used as a digestive aid in the breakdown of protein, and there are now many "digestive-enzyme formulas" that routinely include bromelain as one of the key ingredients. Either bromelain alone or the enzyme formulas can be helpful for people who have digestive conditions such as colitis or irritable bowel syndrome (IBS). In addition, we know that incomplete protein breakdown is implicated in immune reactions that lead to inflammatory conditions such as arthritis.

•Injuries. Bromelain's most well-known use is in the treatment of injuries, and it definitely helps to reduce pain and swelling if you have bruises. In one early clinical trial, doctors gave bromelain to 74 boxers who regularly suffered bruising on the face, lips, ears, chest and arms. When bromelain was given four times a day, all signs of bruising disappeared by the fourth day among 58 of the boxers.

A control group, comprised of 72 boxers, were given a placebo—a look-alike capsule made up of inert substances. In that group, 62 of the boxers needed 7 to 14 days before the bruises cleared up. (Only 10 were free from signs of bruising after 4 days.)

•Respiratory mucus. Bromelain thins mucus. If you have bronchitis and another kind of respiratory-tract condition, you'll probably discover that dosing with bromelain will help you expel the mucus more easily. For similar reasons, taking bromelain has been shown to improve cases of sinusitis.

•Surgery recovery. Bromelain is a valuable supplement in helping people recover more quickly from surgery.

In one study, patients who were given bromelain supplements two to four days before surgery were able to recover from pain and inflammation more quickly than those who didn't take the enzyme. The bromelain-takers took an average of 1.5 days to be pain free, compared with an average of 3.5 days for those who went without it. Without bromelain, it took an average of 6.9 days for inflammation to go down, but only about 2 days for those who had bromelain supplements.

In my opinion, supplements such as bromelain should be routinely given to those recovering from surgery. Just think of all the days of suffering patients could avoid!

•Thrombophlebitis. In studies, bromelain has been proven very effective in the treatment of vein clots, as thrombophlebitis is commonly called.

•Varicose veins. Bromelain has value in the treatment of varicose veins. I do not rate it so effective as horse chestnut and some of the other herbs, but it certainly helps.

Cut Back on Milk

I like a milk shake as much as anyone, but cow's milk is not the wonder food it has been promoted to be.

What's bad about cow's milk? First, tens of millions of Americans are lactose intolerant—they have difficulty digesting the milk sugar *lactose.* Symptoms include nausea, cramps, bloating, gas and/or diarrhea. A lactose-free milk, such as Lactaid, solves this problem, but many other people also react badly to *casein*, a major protein in cow's milk that is also found in Lactaid. This can cause digestive upset, skin rashes, mucous buildup in the sinuses and immune system weakness. Pasteurization destroys enzymes in milk, which makes it harder for *everyone* to digest. And organic milk doesn't sidestep any of the problems listed above.

You can be tested for lactose and casein intolerance—for lactose, you consume some lactose and your breath is tested...for casein, your blood is tested. You also can just stop drinking milk or using it on cereal and see if you feel better. Should you avoid cheese and other dairy products? Maybe—but start with milk and see how it goes.

Consider trying one of the plant-based milks available, such as almond, oat, hazelnut, soy and rice. Many are enriched with such vitamins as D and B-12 as well as calcium—important nutrients in cow's milk.

Peppermint Oil Eases Irritable Bowel Syndrome (IBS)

IBS is a chronic digestive disorder that can cause abdominal pain and bloating...diarrhea or constipation...and urgent, painful, gassy and/or incomplete defecation. In a recent Italian study, 57 IBS patients were given 450 mg of peppermint oil capsules twice daily or a placebo.

Results: Compared with patients taking a placebo, those who took peppermint oil had significantly fewer and milder symptoms at the end of the four-week study and four weeks after therapy was discontinued.

My view: Previous studies showed that peppermint oil relieves IBS symptoms, and now we know that improvement can be achieved in four weeks. Use *enteric-coated* capsules, which pass through the stomach, then dissolve in the small intestine to allow for direct antispasmodic and gas-relieving effects. They are sold in health-food stores and generally are safe. Take 450 mg one hour before breakfast and dinner.

Rhus Toxicodendron— A Soother for Arthritis And Shingles

Rhus toxicodendron (pronounced *roos tox-ih-ko-DEN-dron*) is the homeopathic dilution of poison oak. We know this as a plant that causes a nasty, blistering rash. However, this homeopathic is one of the best skin remedies for relieving symptoms in people who have touched poison ivy. It is also effective in treating eczema, where the skin is very itchy and feels better after the application of very hot water.

I have also used this for people with shingles. The itching, burning pain of the shingles blisters can be relieved in a few days with rhus tox.

Dosage: The typical dosage for rhus tox is 30C potency taken two to three times daily for a day or two for conditions such as stiffness from overexertion. For long-term use for eczema or arthritis, I generally start with a lower dose such as 6C taken two to three times daily.

What are the side effects?: While rhus tox has few side effects, some people may experience skin irritation. People with chronic eczema or arthritis may experience a flare-up of their condition at the beginning of treatment. This is usually a sign that the remedy is working (known as a healing aggravation).

If you do have a flare-up and you begin taking the rhus tox less frequently, you'll probably notice that the flare-up subsides. Soon after, you'll probably notice an improvement in your condition.

If you are not sure whether you should use rhus tox, consult a homeopathic practitioner.

Recommendations for…

•**Arthritis.** Rhus tox is commonly used for osteoarthritis and rheumatoid arthritis. This is probably the right remedy for you if you notice certain characteristics about your symptoms— they are worse in the morning, improve with motion and activity during the day and then get worse again at night while in bed.

Rhus tox is also a good remedy if these arthritic symptoms flare up before a storm or in damp weather. It's probably the right remedy for you if hot baths and showers also provide joint pain relief.

•**Flu.** Rhus tox is a good remedy for the type of flu that makes your joints and muscles stiff.

•**Herpes.** Cold sores on the mouth or face, or genital herpes outbreaks can be helped greatly with rhus tox.

•**Shingles.** This dormant chicken-pox virus erupts when the immune system is weakened. Many elderly people suffer from excruciating pain that is often not relieved with conventional medicines. Rhus tox has worked wonders in several cases I have treated.

•**Strains.** Rhus tox should be used when ligaments and tendons are strained. It helps speed up the recovery process. Athletes should have a supply of rhus tox available at all times.

•**Urticaria.** Urticaria is a fancy way of saying hives. For hive breakouts that do not require emergency treatment (such as when the throat closes), rhus tox helps to relieve the itching and works to heal the lesions more quickly. It is also effective for relieving itching caused by mosquito bites.

The Many Helpful Uses of Zinc

Zinc is a mineral with many important functions. Found in all the cells of the body, it's known as a cofactor—that is, a substance required for numerous enzymatic reactions, including detoxification.

It is important for the synthesis and activity of many hormones such as thymic hormone, growth hormone and insulin, as well as testosterone and other sex hormones. It is necessary for proper immune function and wound healing. It is also needed for protein and DNA synthesis.

Zinc is needed for proper vitamin A metabolism. It is involved in bone formation and in taste.

There are several reasons why people may develop zinc deficiencies. Poor dietary intake is one reason. For example, vegetarians may be more prone to zinc deficiency, as zinc in plant foods is not so bioavailable as in animal products.

Other factors come into play such as genetic susceptibility and some problems with absorption. We also know that certain medications, such as ACE inhibitors like captopril, enalapril and lisinopril that are commonly used to lower blood pressure, can cause zinc deficiency. Other problematic drugs are aspirin and the birth-control pill.

The elderly are more prone to a deficiency because digestive powers decrease as we age, and our bodies don't absorb zinc so well. Alcoholics are at risk for zinc deficiency, and so is anyone with a metabolic disease such as diabetes. When people have diseases of the digestive tract such as Crohn's disease or Celiac disease, and just have general malabsorption—caused by leaky gut syndrome, for instance—they may have impaired mineral absorption.

WHEN ZINC IS MISSING...

Severe nutritional deficiencies are not that common—but I often see people who have marginal or subclinical deficiencies. *Symptoms and conditions associated with zinc deficiency include the following...*

- **Poor wound healing**
- **Lowered immunity; susceptibility to infections**
- **Poor skin and nail health (nails may have white spots)**
- **Fatigue**
- **Loss of taste and smell**
- **Poor growth and development**
- **Blood sugar imbalance**
- **Anorexia; reduced appetite**
- **Delayed sexual development and maturation**
- **Night blindness (due to involvement with vitamin A metabolism)**
- **Infertility**
- **Skin abnormalities**
- **Dandruff**
- **Impaired nerve conduction**
- **Hair loss**
- **Prostate enlargement**
- **Birth malformations**
- **Psychiatric illness**

GETTING YOUR ZINC...

The recommended daily allowance is 15 milligrams per day for adult males and 12 milligrams for adult females. Good food sources include fish and seafood such as oysters and other shellfish. Red meat is also high in zinc.

Eggs and milk also contain ample amounts of zinc. Plant foods such as whole grains and cereals, legumes, nuts and seeds (particularly pumpkin seeds) contain good amounts of zinc, but the mineral isn't so bioavailable as the zinc that comes from animal products.

Breast milk contains a good supply of zinc, so infants are well protected.

Dosage: Adults can benefit from supplementing with an extra 15 to 30 milligrams daily of zinc. Most high-potency multivitamins contain this amount.

Children under one year of age can use a pediatric multivitamin that contains up to 5 milligrams. Children over the age of one can take a children's multivitamin that contains 5 to 15 milligrams in each daily dose.

For specific conditions, such as wound healing or acne, higher dosages of up to 100 milligrams daily may be required for a limited amount of time.

Avoid the use of zinc sulfate, which is not readily absorbed. I recommend other formulas such as zinc picolinate, zinc monomethionine, zinc citrate and zinc chelate.

Note: If you are taking a calcium supplement, take it at a different time from when you take your zinc supplement. The calcium may hinder zinc absorption.

What are the side effects?: Zinc is actually quite a safe supplement, though some people may experience digestive upset if they take zinc on an empty stomach.

High dosages of 150 to 200 milligrams or more, taken over a long period of time, might cause depressed immunity. But I don't recommend taking such high doses anyway, even if you're treating a condition such as severe acne.

One concern is the possibility of developing copper anemia if you are taking high dosages of zinc without taking copper. In the absence of copper, red blood cells change shape; when that happens, they don't carry oxygen so efficiently.

Recommendations from the Natural Physician for…

•**Acne.** Zinc is involved in the metabolism of testosterone. As that "male hormone" is metabolized, it is converted to a metabolite hormone known as DHT (dihydrotestosterone). High levels of DHT are associated with the development of acne, because it increases sebum production. Zinc works to reduce the conversion and also promotes skin healing. Many studies have shown that zinc is beneficial for acne treatment, and at least one indicated that zinc is as effective as tetracycline.

•**AIDS.** People with AIDS are prone to several nutritional deficiencies. Zinc is one of the critical minerals for the immune system, therefore an essential supplement if you have AIDS.

•**Alzheimer's disease.** Zinc may be helpful in slowing the progression of Alzheimer's disease. In a study that included ten people who had Alzheimer's, researchers found that supplementation with zinc helped eight of the people improve memory and communication.

•**Atherosclerosis.** Zinc appears to be one of the many nutrients that helps to prevent atherosclerosis.

•**Birth complications.** Zinc is important during pregnancy because it is required for cell division. A deficiency of zinc is linked to conditions such as premature birth, low birth weight, growth retardation and preeclampsia. A good prenatal multivitamin should help prevent a zinc deficiency when used in combination with a balanced diet.

•**Burns, cuts and wounds.** Zinc is needed for cell division and protein synthesis, both of which are required for skin and wound healing. Burns, cuts and other skin traumas can be relieved with zinc supplements. By taking supplements, you can also speed healing.

•**Common cold.** Several studies have shown that zinc lozenges reduce the severity and duration of the common cold, and also help to relieve sore throats that accompany a cold. It is helpful to take zinc lozenges containing 15 to 25 milligrams of elemental zinc at the first signs of a cold. I find they are particularly good for healing a sore throat.

•**Eating disorders.** Zinc is involved in producing stomach acid as well as stimulating a normal appetite. Studies have shown that people with anorexia and bulimia have deficient zinc levels and may benefit from zinc supplements. Holistic practitioners recommend zinc as part of a comprehensive protocol for people with these eating disorders.

•**Macular degeneration.** Zinc is important in maintaining normal vision. One study of 155 people with macular degeneration found that 45 milligrams of zinc per day significantly slowed the rate of visual loss.

The macula is the portion of the eye that is responsible for fine vision, and when there's degeneration in that area, the sight begins to go. In fact, macular degeneration is the leading cause of blindness in the aged. There are two main types—dry and wet. Nutritional therapy is mainly used for the dry type.

I usually recommend combining zinc supplementation with other important supplements including vitamin C, selenium, carotenoids, taurine, lutein and the herbs ginkgo and bilberry.

•**Male infertility.** Men who are deficient in zinc may have decreased testosterone and sperm production. Studies have shown that zinc supplements increase sperm counts and testosterone in men who previously had deficiencies that prevented conception.

In one study, 11 men who were infertile were treated with 55 milligrams of zinc daily for 6 to 12 months. They showed an increase in sperm count and motility—and three of the men's wives became pregnant during the study.

•**Prostate enlargement.** Zinc is an effective treatment for prostate enlargement. The mineral inhibits the enzyme 5-alpha reductase, which converts testosterone to dihydrotestosterone (DHT). Since high levels of DHT are believed to promote prostate enlargement, I generally prescribe 90 to 100 milligrams daily for men with this condition. After two months, I recommend reducing the zinc dosage to a maintenance level of 50 milligrams.

•**Wilson's disease.** Zinc is one of the primary treatments for this genetic disease in which copper accumulates in the liver and body, causing brain damage. High doses of zinc help to hinder copper absorption.

Get Rid of Your Back Pain Forever

If you've tried everything and still aren't getting relief from back pain, take a lesson from a professional golfer. Two years prior to seeing me, he was ranked in the world's Top 50 golfers and on the PGA's Top 20 earnings list. He was on top of the world—until his back started bothering him.

At first, he thought nothing of it—merely employing ice and heat packs and popping Advil, but the pain wouldn't subside. It got so intense that he started dropping out of events or stopping in the middle of tournaments.

He went to the top sports doctors in the country. He saw orthopedic surgeons, chiropractors, physiatrists (MDs who do physical therapy) and acupuncturists. He had x-rays, CT scans, and MRIs.

They all yielded the same answer: There was nothing structurally wrong with his back— no narrowed discs, torn muscles, sprained ligaments—none of the usual causes of back pain from sports injury.

Determined to "tough it out," he continued playing while taking painkillers, going for chiropractic adjustments, and even getting injections. Nothing helped. The pain got worse and worse, and so did his ability to play golf. His scores suffered, and he went from playing 30 events per year to just 8. Within a few months, the pain became so excruciating that he couldn't even swing a club. Reluctantly, he dropped off the tour, and it looked like his career was over.

Then a friend told him about my clinic. I sensed his exasperation, but the more he described his mysterious ailment, the more confident I became that I could help him. He exhibited the classic symptoms of a hormonal imbalance—specifically a deficiency in *cortisol* (produced by the adrenal glands).

Cortisol is best known as the hormone your body makes under stress, but cortisol is much more. One of its primary tasks is to regulate inflammation. If you don't have enough cortisol, inflammation can escalate to cause immense pain.

WHAT CAUSES CORTISOL DEFICIENCY?

With today's go-go lifestyle, people are under constant stress, so their adrenal glands must work overtime to pump more hormones. Strong glands produce plenty of cortisol, but when adrenals become fatigued from too much stress, cortisol production decreases. Day after day, month after month, year after year, the adrenal glands can weaken.

Low cortisol levels are often accompanied by a deficiency in other hormones produced by the adrenals, such as DHEA. It's instrumental in helping your body heal from injuries, like the microscopic muscle tears you would get from repeatedly swinging a golf club! The good news is that in the vast majority of cases, adrenal fatigue is not permanent, and neither is the back pain it causes. Simply take the proper remedies to strengthen your glands and give them time to rest and rebuild.

So what happened to the golfer? After confirming the diagnosis with tests, I prescribed the herbs rhodiola and Siberian ginseng, plus some glandular extracts. I also put him on low-dose DHEA and minute doses of cortisol to take some strain off of his glands and regulate his hormonal levels while his adrenals healed. Within a few days, he was reporting less pain. Six weeks later, he was practicing again, and three months later, he made his comeback—playing in two PGA tournaments back-to-back!

His story is dramatic, but by no means unique. You don't have to be a famous athlete to suffer from adrenal fatigue; I've successfully treated well over a thousand patients—primarily age fifty and over. So if your back pain's resistant to the usual treatments, have your cortisol and DHEA levels checked. *If standard saliva, blood or urine tests indicate deficiencies, discuss the following remedies with your practitioner…*

•**Rhodiola Rosea**—500 mg—standardized to contain 3% to 5% rosavins—twice daily before meals.

•**Adrenal Glandular Extract**—250 mg, two-to-three times daily, before meals.

•**Ashwagandha**—250 to 500 mg of a standardized product daily before meals

•**Pantothenic Acid**—500 mg, three times daily with meals, along with a 50 mg B-complex or multi-supplement containing the remaining B vitamins.

•**Vitamin C**—1000 to 2000 mg twice daily.

•**DHEA**—5 to 15 mg for women, or 15 to 25 mg for men, daily with breakfast.

•**Cortisol**—2.5 to 5 mg three-to-four times daily.

Proven Health Benefits of Spirituality and Prayer

Marty Sullivan, MD, associate professor of medicine and former director of science and healing, Center for Integrated Medicine at Duke University School of Medicine, Durham, NC.

Marty Sullivan, MD, a leading expert on integrative medicine, talks about the connection between spirituality and health.

•**In what ways does spirituality make a person healthier?** People with strong spiritual beliefs tend to live longer. They are less likely to develop heart disease, cancer and other serious illnesses. They are more energetic and less likely to feel depressed or anxious.

Some studies have shown spiritual beliefs to be more important for good health than not smoking. That's a striking finding.

•**How does spirituality reduce stress?** People who pray or meditate experience the relaxation response—a drop in blood pressure, heart rate and levels of stress hormones, such as cortisol.

Prayer and meditation also cause an increase in alpha and theta waves. These electrical impulses in the brain are associated with relaxation.

Even if you do not pray or meditate, having religious or spiritual beliefs can reduce anxiety and increase levels of interleukin-6, a blood protein that indicates good immune function.

One theory is that the social support from spiritual communities—such as churches, meditation groups or yoga classes—helps people buffer the harmful effects of stress.

Of course, people with strong religious feelings believe that God is the healing force.

Not all spiritual beliefs are equally beneficial. People with positive spiritual beliefs—such as the idea that God represents love and forgiveness—do better than those who believe in harsh divine punishment.

•**Can praying for someone to get well speed his/her recovery?** Many studies have explored the concept of distance healing. One study looked at AIDS patients. Over a period of one year, those who were prayed for were 70% less likely to develop AIDS-related illnesses or other complications than those who were not prayed for.

•**Is it possible that prayer has a placebo effect—that it works only because people think it will?** In most of the studies, neither the patients nor the doctors knew who was being prayed for. That rules out any placebo effect.

Prayer can even affect the growth of yeast and other laboratory organisms. Obviously, these are not affected by the power of positive thinking.

•**How can we increase our own spirituality?** Set aside 20 minutes for quiet time daily. Spend it meditating...listening to music...or simply allowing yourself to think about the wonders of nature, a memorable line from a poem, etc.

Read spiritual books, poetry or essays. People who practice formal religion often turn to classic texts, such as the Bible. Others might be interested in reading the works of philosophers or theologians.

Be part of a spiritual community. If you don't attend a church or temple, consider taking meditation or yoga classes...or going on spiritual retreats.

Give to others. Nearly all of the world's religions and spiritual traditions emphasize charitable giving. When you share with others, you form deeper connections with a world that is greater than yourself.

Melatonin Reduces Blood Pressure

A randomized, double-blind study involved 18 women, ages 47 to 63, half with hypertension being successfully controlled with ACE inhibitor medication and half who had normal blood pressure. For three weeks, participants took either 3 mg of time-released melatonin (a supplement typically used to promote sleep) or a placebo one hour before bed. They were then switched to the other treatment for another three weeks. After taking melatonin for three weeks, 84% of the women had at least a 10 mm/Hg decrease in nocturnal (nighttime) systolic and diastolic blood pressure, while only 39% experienced a decrease in nocturnal blood pressure after taking the placebo. The reduction was the greatest in those with controlled hypertension. In both groups, no change was found in daytime blood pressure readings. Previous studies have found similar results when men with untreated hypertension took melatonin.

My view: Melatonin, a hormone produced by the pineal gland in the brain, is secreted in response to darkness and promotes a normal sleep cycle. A deficiency of melatonin may prevent relaxation of the cardiovascular and nervous systems, increasing blood pressure. (Normally, heart rate and blood vessel constriction decrease at night.) While people with hypertension often monitor their daytime blood pressure, they usually are unaware of their readings at night. This can be a mistake. High nighttime blood pressure is just as important as high daytime pressure. For people with high blood pressure whose levels also tend to be elevated at night, I recommend taking 3 mg of time-released melatonin one hour before bed. To determine if you have elevated blood pressure at night, use a home blood pressure monitor to test levels several times during the day and twice a night (at midnight and 4:00 am) for three days.

Caution: Consult your doctor before trying melatonin. It may require an adjustment to your blood pressure medication. Women who are pregnant or breastfeeding, as well as those taking birth control pills, should not use melatonin.

A Homeopathic Remedy For Bruises

The homeopathic remedy *Arnica montana* (also known as leopard's bane), significantly reduces bruising. In a double-blind clinical trial involving 29 women who were undergoing face-lifts, participants were randomly assigned to receive homeopathic arnica (12C potency) or a placebo beginning the morning of surgery. The treatment was repeated every eight hours for four days. Facial bruising and swelling were evaluated by doctors and nurses, as well as through a computerized digital-image analysis of photographs taken before and after surgery. Subjective symptoms—those observed by the patients and professional staff—and the degree of discoloration were not significantly improved by the arnica. However, the area of bruising was significantly smaller for the group of subjects who took arnica. Although the study was on women, I would expect the same results for men and for other types of bruising.

Arnica preparations have been used in homeopathic medicine for two centuries. *Sesquiterpene lactones,* major active compounds in arnica, are known to reduce inflammation, decrease pain and improve circulation.

I can attest to hundreds of cases in which arnica has reduced pain and swelling. I also have seen this benefit with infants and animals—where a placebo effect is unlikely. You can use arnica for any soft-tissue injury, such as bruising after a fall or a sprained ankle. The most common dose is two pellets of 30C strength taken two to four times daily for two days. Or apply homeopathic arnica cream two to three times daily until healed. Arnica is sold at most health-food stores and some pharmacies.

Caution: Do not use topical arnica on broken skin or open wounds.

Hyaluronic Acid

On her first visit to me, 60-year-old Jenny said, "Every time I hear of a supplement that might reduce my arthritis pain, I try it—but I've gotten very little relief. I've almost given up on finding anything that works." I paid close attention as she named nearly a dozen supplements she had taken for the arthritis in her hips and knees. Then I mentioned one oral supplement that had not been on her list—*hyaluronic acid* (HA). "I've never even heard of it, but it's worth trying," Jenny said. Six weeks later, she walked nimbly into my clinic and reported a dramatic reduction in her pain and stiffness. She was surprised at this success—but I was not.

HA has been so effective for so many of my arthritis patients that I consider it an up-and-coming superstar among nutritional supplements.

Bonus: HA also promotes skin health.

WHAT IS HYALURONIC ACID?

A naturally occurring substance in the body, the HA molecule is formed by two sugars strung together in a long chain. HA is an essential component of the joints, skin, eyes and blood vessels (as well as the umbilical cord). HA deficiencies, which develop for reasons that are not well-understood, contribute to premature aging and disease in these tissues. As yet, there is no reliable test to measure HA levels.

HA is a key component of *synovial fluid,* the lubricating fluid in joint cavities. This fluid, which is secreted by a membrane that forms a capsule around the ends of bones, has two main purposes. First, it helps to minimize friction and prevent breakdown of the joints (like the oil used to lubricate moving car parts). Second, synovial fluid helps with shock absorption within joints. Cartilage is the main shock absorber, but it does not contain blood vessels—so synovial fluid transports the nutrients required for cartilage healing and regeneration, and removes waste products. In addition, HA is an actual component of cartilage and is required for healthy cartilage formation.

There are two main types of arthritis. *Osteoarthritis* is caused by the normal wear and tear of aging and/or by injury. *Rheumatoid arthritis* is an autoimmune disease in which the immune system attacks the body's own joint tissue and causes deterioration. As either type of arthritis progresses, the synovial fluid degrades, lessening its lubricating and shock-absorbing abilities...and cartilage breaks down and becomes

inflamed. Supplementing with HA helps to counteract both of these effects.

THE FIGHT AGAINST ARTHRITIS

When I mention HA to patients, most say they've never heard of it. I expect this to change as news of HA's effectiveness spreads.

•**HA injections.** In 1997, HA injections were approved by the FDA for patients with osteoarthritis of the knee, and they now are being studied for use in shoulder, hip and ankle joints. Injectable HA products include Hyalgan, Supartz, Orthovisc and Synvisc.

HA injections go directly into the affected joint or joints...are done in a doctor's office using local anesthetic...take just a few minutes...and usually are given three to five times, each one week apart. Side effects include minor swelling, temporary pain, rash and/or bruising at the injection site. While not everyone who receives HA injections finds relief, for many people the painful symptoms of arthritis are noticeably reduced for up to six months (especially in the early stages of the disease), allowing patients to delay or avoid joint-replacement surgery.

For now, only a limited number of rheumatologists and osteopaths provide this therapy. HA shots cost about $230 each and may or may not be covered by insurance, depending on your policy. Fortunately, there is a promising alternative —oral HA.

•**HA oral supplementation.** With regard to HA's use as an oral supplement, the big question is whether it can be absorbed and used by the body when taken in capsule form. Critics of HA supplementation say that its molecular structure is too large to be absorbed in the digestive tract—yet several studies in the past four years have shown otherwise.

One of the first studies to demonstrate that HA is absorbed effectively into the bloodstream and the joints was presented at the 2004 Experimental Biology Conference. Researchers gave rats and dogs one oral dose of HA that was *radio labeled* (chemically joined with a radioactive substance), allowing it to be tracked with diagnostic imaging.

Result: HA was absorbed into the animals' bloodstreams and distributed to their joints. Although no similar studies have been done on people, I think it is logical to assume that HA's absorbability in humans may be similar to its action in animals.

Why am I keen on supplemental HA for arthritis? During the past year, several dozens of my patients with osteoarthritis and rheumatoid arthritis have taken nonprescription oral HA with good results. I have found that HA by itself can produce significant results—and in many cases, results are even better when HA is taken in combination with mainstay joint supplements, such as chondroitin, fish oil, glucosamine, *methylsulfonylmethane* (MSM) and/or *S-adenosylmethionine* (SAMe).

This is wonderful news, because HA often allows patients to reduce or discontinue pharmaceutical nonsteroidal anti-inflammatory (NSAID) drugs, such as *ibuprofen* (Motrin) and *naproxen* (Aleve). These drugs are associated with serious adverse side effects, including bleeding stomach ulcers, liver and kidney damage and increased risk for heart attack and stroke.

HA is an example of a supplement that works well in the real world but has generated limited published data. Existing research mostly involves a patented HA product called BioCell Collagen II (714-632-1231, *www.biocelltechnology.com*), made from the sternal cartilage of chickens and used as an ingredient in various brands of HA oral supplements. One small study included 16 patients with osteoarthritis of the knee or hand who were taking COX-2 inhibitors or other NSAIDs. Eight patients took 1,000 mg of BioCell daily, while the other eight took a placebo. After two months of treatment, the group receiving BioCell reported significant improvement in pain, range of motion and swelling—whereas the placebo group showed no significant changes. One such product, sold at health-food stores, is BioCell Chicken Sternum Collagen Type II, made by Premier Labs (800-887-5227, *www.premierlabs.com*).

Other oral products contain a type of HA called *sodium hyaluronate,* which is produced during microbial fermentation. While I am not aware of any human studies on this form of HA, animal studies suggest that it is safe and several of my patients have reported positive effects. One such product available in health-food stores is Now Foods Hyaluronic Acid (888-669-3663, *www.nowfoods.com*). The recommended dosage is 100 mg twice daily. The Now Foods capsules, like brands that contain BioCell, can be used indefinitely, generally are safe and only rarely cause mild digestive upset.

HYALURONIC HELP FOR THE SKIN

Another benefit of HA is that it improves the health of the largest human organ—the skin. *Here's how…*

One of the most important proteins of the skin is collagen, the "glue" of connective tissue that holds the skin together, thereby maintaining its elasticity and form. HA supports collagen production and also is critical for maintaining moisture in and between skin cells. A lack of HA—typically brought on by illness or aging—may contribute to skin dryness, thinning and wrinkles.

•**HA injections.** Like the better-known collagen injections, HA injections can be used to minimize wrinkles, lines and pitting from acne or scars, and to plump up thin lips. HA and collagen injections both typically need to be repeated after six to nine months—but HA is less likely to provoke an allergic reaction.

FDA-approved HA injectable skin fillers include Hylaform and Restylane. Possible side effects include brief redness, swelling and/or tenderness at the injection site. Health insurance generally does not cover cosmetic treatments.

Caution: Cosmetic HA injections should be administered by an experienced cosmetic surgeon, not a family practitioner.

•**HA oral supplementation.** Recently I spoke with a patient who had thin, easily bruised skin as a result of using oral steroids for several years to treat Crohn's disease (an inflammatory condition of the digestive tract). After various foods and supplements failed to improve her skin condition, I recommended an HA oral supplement called Purity Products Ultimate HA Formula (888-769-7873, *www.purityproducts.com*). Eight weeks after she started to take HA, this patient reported that for the first time in years, she was not covered in bruises.

Note: HA oral supplements designed to promote skin health generally contain the same active HA ingredient as those marketed for joint health.

•**HA topical ointment.** Some evidence suggests that HA skin ointment also may reduce wrinkles and skin pitting. One study I obtained from a private research lab showed that topical HA inhibited production of *hyaluronidase,* an enzyme in the skin and connective tissues that degrades the body's own natural wrinkle-fighting HA. In a separate *in vitro* (test-tube) study from Pennsylvania State University, topical HA was shown to stimulate production of collagen-producing cells called *fibroblasts,* which potentially could further reduce wrinkles and lines.

One commercially available topical skin product that contains BioCell is Skin Eternal Hyaluronic Serum by Source Naturals (800-815-2333, *www. sourcenaturals.com*). Place one to four drops of serum on your finger and gently massage into the skin where desired. It is generally safe for everyone. Rare side effects may include redness and irritation. I suggest trying it for two months to evaluate its effectiveness. If you are satisfied, topical HA can be used indefinitely to optimize the health and appearance of your skin.

While further studies clearly are needed to confirm the benefits of HA, I am optimistic about its potential. After all, it is not often that so promising a therapy arrives on the health-care scene.

FURTHER RELIEF FROM ARTHRITIS

For maximum relief from arthritis pain and inflammation, combine HA oral supplements or injections with other natural supplements described below. All are available in health-food stores and, unless noted, generally are safe for everyone. Mild arthritis symptoms may respond to the lower end of the dosage range, while severe symptoms may require the higher dosage.

•**Chondroitin,** a substance derived from cow cartilage.

Dosage: 1,200 mg daily. Lower the dosage or discontinue use if you experience digestive upset, such as nausea.

•**Fish oil** in the form of *docosahexaenoic acid* (DHA) and *eicosapentaenoic acid* (EPA), combined.

Dosage: 1,000 mg to 2,000 mg daily.

Caution: Get your doctor's approval first if you take a blood thinner, such as aspirin or *warfarin* (Coumadin).

•**Glucosamine,** a substance derived from shellfish.

Dosage: 1,500 mg daily. Lower the dosage or discontinue use if you experience digestive upset, such as diarrhea.

Caution: Check with your doctor before using if you are allergic to shellfish...or if you have diabetes, because glucosamine may cause blood-sugar fluctuations.

•**Methylsulfonylmethane (MSM),** an organic sulfur compound.

Dosage: 2,000 mg to 6,000 mg daily.

•**S-adenosylmethionine (SAMe),** an amino acid-like substance.

Dosage: 600 mg to 1,200 mg daily.

How to use: For rheumatoid arthritis, take fish oil and MSM. For osteoarthritis, start with glucosamine and MSM...and if symptoms are not adequately relieved within two months, also take chondroitin, fish oil and SAMe.

Back Pain Relief

Picking up a heavy box, you get a sudden stab of pain in your lower back—and now all you feel like doing is lying down. Or while sitting at your desk, you rub your aching back, thinking resignedly that it's time for surgery. If these scenarios sound familiar, don't be too hasty to follow through—or you may regret it.

Now we know: Bed rest for lower back pain (LBP) may do more harm than good...and surgery, once routine for certain lower back problems, is usually unnecessary.

LBP can result from an injury to muscles, tendons and/or ligaments that surround the spine. Or the problem can occur in the spine itself—for instance, misaligned vertebrae or a herniated disc (when the gel-like inner pulp of the disc between two vertebrae bulges out and irritates nearby nerves). Less frequently, LBP is due to nerve damage from an infection or tumor, osteoporosis (brittle bones) or problems with the kidneys or other organs.

LBP is called acute if it lasts several days to several weeks...and chronic if it lasts a few months or more. Acute LBP typically comes on suddenly, when an abrupt twist of the body or an attempt to lift something heavy leads to a muscle strain or spasm. Acute pain may ease quickly as the tissues heal, or it may persist due to tiny tears in the muscle and become chronic. When LBP is caused by a spine problem, discomfort usually grows as the condition gradually worsens. If back pain is severe or lasts for more than a week, see your doctor or a physiatrist (a physician specializing in musculoskeletal health). Typically the cause of LBP can be determined by a physical exam, X-ray and/or MRI.

PAIN RELIEF RIGHT NOW

Doctors used to think that the best treatment for acute LBP was strict bed rest—and this belief persists among the general population, though many studies show that bed rest delays recovery. Obviously, you should avoid exercising or lifting until pain eases significantly, but do not try to remain motionless.

To reduce pain and inflammation, apply a cold pack to the sore area for about 15 minutes out of each waking hour. After 24 hours, alternate the hourly 15-minute applications between cold and heat. Heat relaxes muscles and increases blood flow to the area. Continue until pain subsides.

Convenient: Instant single-use heat and cold packs that self-activate...or reusable microwavable heat packs and freezable cold packs (both sold at drugstores).

Also, consult a chiropractor for *spinal manipulation*—hands-on maneuvers that stretch and realign the spine and surrounding tissues, relieving pain.

Evidence: A study in the *Journal of Manipulative and Physiological Therapeutics* compared 93 LBP patients treated by chiropractors with 45 patients treated by family physicians. After one month, 56% of the chiropractic group felt better or much better, but only 13% of the other group experienced such improvement. To find a practitioner, contact the American Chiropractic Association (703-276-8800, *www.amerchiro. org*). If you have *spinal stenosis* (narrowing of the spinal canal), do not have spinal manipulation—it could damage the spinal cord.

In addition, consider acupuncture, which reduces muscle spasms and releases natural painkillers called *endorphins*...massage therapy, which relaxes tight muscles and increases blood flow to the sore area...and/or physical therapy,

which uses exercises, hands-on maneuvers, heat and cold to promote healing.

SOOTHING SUPPLEMENTS

Various natural substances can alleviate back pain. All are sold at health-food stores and, unless otherwise noted, generally are safe and can be taken until symptoms are gone. Use the lower end of each dosage range if you weigh less than 200 pounds, and the higher dosage if you weigh more or if relief has not been achieved within one week. Depending on the aggressiveness of the treatment you desire, these supplements can be used individually, in any combination or even all together.

To reduce muscle pain and inflammation...

•**Devil's claw,** an African root.

Dosage: For acute pain, take 800 mg three times daily of concentrated extract capsules (standardized to 1.5% to 3% harpagosides) for up to two weeks. For chronic pain, take 200 mg to 400 mg three times daily for up to eight weeks. Consult a doctor before using if you have diabetes. Do not use if you have an ulcer, heartburn, gastritis or gallstones...are pregnant or nursing...or take a blood thinner, such as aspirin or *warfarin* (Coumadin).

•**Protease (protein-digesting) enzymes.**

Dosage: Bromelain at 1,000 mg three times daily between meals.

Alternative: A combination enzyme formula, such as Wobenzym from Mucos Pharma (866-962-6996, *www.wobenzym-usa.com*). Take five to 10 tablets three times daily on an empty stomach. Do not use if you take a blood thinner or have an ulcer.

•**B vitamins.**

Dosage: Vitamin B-1 and vitamin B-6, each at 50 mg to 100 mg three times daily...plus vitamin B-12 at 250 micrograms (mcg) to 500 mcg three times daily.

To ease muscle spasms...

•**Methylsulfonylmethane (MSM),** an organic sulfur compound.

Dosage: 4,000 mg to 8,000 mg daily.

•**Magnesium.**

Dosage: 250 mg twice daily.

•**Calcium.**

Dosage: 500 mg twice daily.

To alleviate stiffness...

•**Rhus tox,** a homeopathic remedy derived from poison ivy.

Dosage: Two pellets four times daily of a 30C potency.

To soothe nerve pain...

•**St. John's wort oil.** Rub a bean-size amount of this herbal oil over the affected area twice daily.

Natural supplements may take 24 hours or more to provide relief. In the interim, if pain is severe, also take an over-the-counter nonsteroidal anti-inflammatory drug (NSAID), such as aspirin, *ibuprofen* (Advil) or *naproxen* (Aleve). Or ask your doctor about prescription pain medication, such as *hydrocodone with acetaminophen* (Vicodin)...and/or a prescription muscle relaxant, such as *cyclobenzaprine* (Flexeril). Take these medications as briefly as possible to minimize the risk of side effects, such as ulcers, kidney disease and/or liver damage.

LONG-TERM HEALING STRATEGIES

Chronic LBP often results from poor posture, which misaligns the spine and weakens torso muscles. These exercise regimens can help...

•**Alexander Technique** teaches proper body mechanics and movement techniques.

Referrals: American Society for the Alexander Technique (800-473-0620, *www.alexander tech.org*).

•**Feldenkrais Method** is administered as one-on-one manipulation and/or group instruction in proper alignment.

Referrals: Feldenkrais Guild of North America (800-775-2118, *www.feldenkraisguild.com*).

•**Pilates** targets supportive "core" muscles of the torso.

Referrals: Pilates Method Alliance (866-573-4945, *www.pilatesmethodalliance.org*).

•**Yoga** increases flexibility, balance and muscle strength.

Referrals: International Association of Yoga Therapists (928-541-0004, *www.iayt.org*).

Surprisingly, LBP also may result from foot problems that lead to spinal misalignment— such as when arches are too flat or too high (so feet roll inward or outward) or when one leg is slightly shorter than the other. A podiatrist can provide supportive custom-made orthotic shoe inserts that promote proper alignment, allowing back muscles to heal.

WHEN TO CALL 911

Back pain that is accompanied by certain other symptoms can signal a medical emergency.

Heart attack can cause back pain and...

•**Chest pain,** especially if there also is a crushing or squeezing sensation

•**Sweating**

•**Shortness of breath**

•**Nausea**

•**Pain that spreads** into the jaw, shoulders or arms.

Spinal injury can cause back pain and...

•**Weakness in the legs**

•**Numbness or tingling** in the buttocks, genital area or legs

•**Loss of bowel or bladder control.**

If you experience any of these symptoms in conjunction with back pain, call 911 and be specific—"I think I'm having a heart attack" or "I think I have a spinal injury." This is not the time to be stoic about back pain.

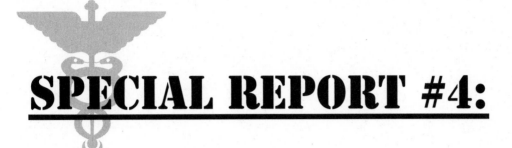

SPECIAL REPORT #4:

Free Cures and
Low-Cost
Home Remedies

Free Cures and Low-Cost Home Remedies

Boost Your Mood Without Drugs

Feeling down? You're not alone. We all have gloomy moments. But if you're chronically feeling sad, apathetic, irritable or "emotionally numb," you could be suffering from chronic depression. It affects one in four women and one in eight men at some time in their lives.

Sadness is perfectly normal if you recently experienced a traumatic event, such as a loved one's death, a divorce or a job loss. Anyone who is going through such a situation should talk about it with family members, friends or a counselor. Some people come to terms with these feelings in just a few weeks. Others require months or even years. Just remember, though, that suppressed grief or anger is a common cause of depression.

If you're feeling particularly down—and everything in your life is basically fine—you could be suffering from depression that has a biochemical basis linked to genetics. If a parent or sibling has experienced depression, your risk increases by two to four times. In these cases, conventional doctors often recommend prescription antidepressants. But all antidepressants have side effects, including fatigue, weight gain, low libido, liver toxicity and/or dizziness.*

WHAT'S BRINGING YOU DOWN?

The study of brain chemistry has led to advances in the treatment of depression. We are learning more about how chemicals that are produced in the body—and even certain foods—affect our moods.

Here's why: You have trillions of nerve cells (neurons) in your nervous system. Signals pass among these cells via chemical messengers

Warning: If you currently are taking an anti-depressant, do not discontinue use without supervision from a doctor. If you have suicidal thoughts, seek immediate medical attention.

Mark A. Stengler, ND, naturopathic physician in private practice, La Jolla, California...adjunct associate clinical professor at the National College of Natural Medicine, Portland, Oregon...author of many books, including *The Natural Physician's Healing Therapies* and coauthor of *Prescription for Natural Cures* (both from Bottom Line Books)...and author of the *Bottom Line/Natural Healing* newsletter.

known as *neurotransmitters*. When neuro-transmitters aren't working properly, your mood, memory and comprehension suffer.

The antidepressants that conventional doctors prescribe aim to restore balance to one or more neurotransmitters artificially. These drugs may improve symptoms of depression, but the trade-off is the risk of side effects.

The natural approach I recommend—focusing on foods and supplements—is a safe, effective way to boost the activity of the neurotransmitters that are key players in mood adjustment…

• **Serotonin,** the "feel-good neurotransmitter," is made by the body from the amino acid *tryptophan,* which is found in such foods as turkey and milk. If your serotonin levels are adequate, you will feel calm, sociable and relaxed much of the time. If you have depression or anxiety, your serotonin levels may be too low.

• **Norepinephrine** is produced when you're under stress, along with the hormone *adrenaline.* A low level of norepinephrine is believed to lead to depression. This neurotransmitter, also known as *noradrenaline,* is made from the amino acid *tyrosine,* which is found in dairy products, meat, fish, wheat and oats.

• **Dopamine** affects motor control (movement of body parts), motivation and your response to reward, such as winning a game or seeing a stock you own go way up. Like norepinephrine, dopamine is made from tyrosine.

• **Gamma-aminobutyric acid** (GABA) has a calming effect on the brain and nervous system. A GABA deficiency is commonly associated with anxiety. This neurotransmitter is made from the amino acids *taurine* (found in meat and fish) and *glutamine* (also found in meat and fish as well as in beans and dairy products).

GET A LIFT FROM OMEGA-3s

Neurotransmitters need nutrients to function properly. One whole class of nutrients required for normal mood and alertness is omega-3 fatty acids—particularly *eicosapentaenoic acid* (EPA) and *docosahexaenoic acid* (DHA), which are found in fish and fish oil and in omega-3–fortified products, such as some eggs. Studies show that people who have low omega-3 levels are more likely to suffer from depression. This is particularly true among older adults. Studies have

confirmed that depression is less prevalent in countries where the population eats a lot of fish.

Regardless of whether you're taking an anti-depressant or a supplement for depression, it's a good idea to eat at least two servings a week of omega-3–rich fish, such as salmon, sardines and trout. In addition, taking fish-oil supplements can be helpful for those prone to depression. Take a product that provides a daily dose of 1,000 mg of combined EPA and DHA. Fish-oil supplements are widely available at health-food stores.

Good brands: Nordic Naturals (800-662-2544, *www.nordicnaturals.com*) and Carlson Laboratories (888-234-5656, *www.carlsonlabs.com*).

CHECK YOUR AMINO ACIDS

Amino acids also are key to a nutrition-based approach to depression. There are 10 amino acids that are absolutely essential but that our bodies can't produce. These amino acids are found in the proteins that we eat and are converted into the neurotransmitters that affect mood. If your diet lacks protein—found in eggs, poultry, meat and fish and, in smaller amounts, in plant foods such as soy, lentils and peanuts—these essential amino acids may be in short supply.

If you suffer from depression, get a blood or urine test that measures your amino acid levels. Tests are available through a holistic or medical doctor's office. Metametrix (800-221-4640, *www.metametrix.com*) is one of several labs that offer this testing through doctors' offices. The test costs $265 and may be covered by insurance. If an amino acid deficiency is detected, you and your doctor can decide how to correct it. Amino Acid Complex 1000 by KAL is a reliable supplement and can be found at most health-food stores.

DON'T FORGET YOUR Bs

Researchers have learned that we need plenty of B vitamins to help activate mood-regulating neuro-transmitters. If you have low levels of B-12 or folic acid—two important B vitamins—you're more likely to be depressed. Deficiencies of vitamins B-1 and B-6 can affect mood as well. B-vitamin deficiencies are especially common among people in their 60s or older. Try to eat foods that are rich in B vitamins, such as whole grains and green, leafy vegetables.

Ask your doctor for a vitamin B-12 and folate blood test if you're a woman who uses oral contraceptives, you frequently consume coffee and/or alcohol or you're under extreme stress. People over age 60 should be tested annually. I advise anyone who has a B-vitamin deficiency to take a 50-mg B-complex vitamin once daily and a full-spectrum multivitamin that includes B vitamins and other important ingredients, such as selenium, inositol, iron and vitamin D. Deficiencies of these nutrients also have been linked to depression.

MOOD-LIFTING SUPPLEMENTS

The following supplements are most effective for treating depression. Start with *5-hydroxytryptophan* (5-HTP). If you don't feel better within a month, add *S-adenosylmethionine* (SAMe) and/or St. John's wort.

•**5-HTP** is made by the body from the amino acid *L-tryptophan* and converted into *serotonin*. The supplement form of 5-HTP—available at health-food stores—is naturally derived from the seeds of the West African plant *Griffonia simplicifolia*. I recommend taking 100 mg two to three times daily on an empty stomach.

Caution: Don't take 5-HTP if you're on an antidepressant, antianxiety or other psychiatric medication. Nursing and pregnant women also should avoid it.

•**SAMe,** a substance that occurs naturally in the body, helps neurotransmitters form efficiently. Studies have shown that it is as effective at reducing depression as prescription antidepressants and produces fewer side effects. In studies, people with depression have taken up to 1,600 mg of SAMe daily, but I have found that most patients benefit from 600 mg to 800 mg taken daily in two divided doses a half-hour before meals. For best results, also take a 50-mg B-complex supplement once daily. SAMe is not recommended if you have manic depression, a disorder characterized by cycles of severe highs (manias) and lows (depression)…if you're on a prescription antidepressant or psychiatric medication…or if you're a woman who is pregnant or nursing.

•**St. John's wort** is an herb that helps treat anxiety and mild-to-moderate depression. Various constituents of St. John's wort flowers and leaves have been shown to stabilize a variety of neurotransmitters, including serotonin, dopamine

and norepinephrine. A study reported in the medical journal *International Clinical Psychopharmacology* found that St. John's wort given for six weeks was as effective as the prescription antidepressant *fluoxetine* (Prozac) in treating depression and caused fewer side effects. I recommend 300 mg daily of an extract containing the active ingredients *hypericin* (0.3%) and *hyperforin* (3% to 5%). Such formulations are available at health-food stores. Side effects are rare, though some people experience mild digestive upset, fatigue, sleep disturbances, itching and skin rash.

Caution: St. John's wort can interact with antidepressants and other psychiatric drugs, so seek a doctor's advice if you are taking any of these medications and want to try this herb.

GET MOVING

Exercise is another underrated treatment and prevention strategy for depression. Researchers at Duke University Medical Center found that patients with clinical depression who exercised regularly were less likely to have a relapse than those who underwent drug therapy only.

Exercise balances stress hormones, activates feel-good brain chemicals known as *endorphins* and improves blood flow to the brain. I recommend 30 to 60 minutes of exercise three times weekly.

STAY CONNECTED

Work with a licensed professional who has experience treating depression to explore possible situations or conditions that trigger your depression.

Avoid isolating yourself—this worsens depression. Research shows that people who maintain strong ties to family members and/or friends are less susceptible to depression.

For some people, proper nutrition and taking supplements don't successfully treat depression. If your symptoms don't improve with the natural therapy I have recommended above, work with your doctor to investigate other possible causes, such as hormone deficiencies, food sensitivities, hypoglycemia (low blood sugar), lack of sunlight (which leads to vitamin D deficiency and seasonal affective disorder, also known as SAD), toxic metals (such as mercury), sleep problems and candidiasis (overgrowth of *Candida albicans* yeast).

Some drugs can lead to depression. Common culprits are steroids, antihistamines, blood pressure medications, anti-inflammatory drugs, narcotics and—believe it or not—antidepressants, such as fluoxetine.

Are You Depressed?

If you have experienced two or more of the following symptoms for two consecutive weeks, you could be suffering from depression…*

•**Persistent sadness, anxiety or "empty" mood.**

•**Feelings of hopelessness, pessimism, guilt or worthlessness.**

•**Loss of interest in activities that you once enjoyed,** including sex.

•**Restlessness, irritability or fatigue.**

•**Difficulty concentrating, remembering or making decisions.**

•**Insomnia, early-morning awakening or oversleeping.**

•**Loss of appetite and weight loss.**

•**Overeating and weight gain.**

•**Physical symptoms that don't respond to treatment,** such as headaches, digestive disorders and chronic pain.

•**Thoughts of death or suicide or suicide attempts.**

*If these symptoms interfere with your ability to function, you may be suffering from clinical depression. A less severe type of chronic depression is dysthymia, which can cause the same symptoms over a period of years but is less disabling.

National Institute of Mental Health

Computers and Eyestrain

How can you relieve eye soreness that results from prolonged computer use? The most important thing is to move your eyes away from the screen every 10 to 15 minutes to give them a break from the glare and relax the eye muscles.

You also can alleviate eyestrain by using the cupping technique several times during the day. To do this, cup your hands over your closed eyes and hold them there for 30 seconds while taking deep breaths to your abdomen—this helps you relax and improves oxygenation.

See page 88 for more help with eyestrain.

Growth Hormone to Fight Aging

For over 15 years, growth hormone (GH) has been touted as a miraculous antiaging hormone. Some physicians also prescribe it for obesity, sexual dysfunction, cognitive decline and fibromyalgia. Even some healthy athletes and bodybuilders use GH.

WHAT IS GROWTH HORMONE?

GH is secreted by the brain's pituitary gland. As its name implies, it stimulates the growth of tissues in the body. Most notably, it promotes growth in height during childhood. Most people have heard of a childhood deficiency of GH, but in rare cases, adults can lack adequate amounts of the hormone. A GH deficiency that occurs during adulthood can lead to a reduction in muscle mass, strength and bone density as well as sexual dysfunction and emotional problems, such as depression. If you have these symptoms, ask your doctor for a blood test. A GH deficiency even can increase cardiovascular disease risk.

THE ANTIAGING CRAZE

In 1990, the *New England Journal of Medicine* reported on a six-month study in which 12 healthy men, ages 61 to 81, who showed no signs of GH deficiency were given twice the dose of GH that an adult man with a deficiency would ordinarily receive. A control group of nine men did not receive GH injections. The men receiving the injections experienced systolic (top number) blood pressure and fasting blood glucose concentrations that were significantly higher than when they started the study. On the positive side, they experienced an increase in lean body mass, a decrease in fat mass and an improvement in bone density, all of which led many people to believe that GH could be used to effectively reverse some of these troubling signs of aging. However, there have been no studies of GH's effect on longevity in humans.

SAFETY CONCERNS

I have tested many patients' blood levels of insulinlike growth factor (IGF-1)—a biomarker that is used to assess GH levels. Only occasionally have I found a patient with a serious deficiency. Typically, these patients suffer from fatigue. What concerns me is that some doctors routinely recommend GH injections for virtually all of their patients who are over age 60 without testing for a deficiency. When these doctors do run blood tests, they often diagnose a deficiency by comparing their older patients' IGF-1 levels with those of a 20-year-old. I strongly disagree with this practice. GH should not be used unnecessarily because of the side effects, which include blurred vision, burning or tingling in the legs and arms, dizziness, severe headache, back pain, chills, difficulty breathing, fever, hair loss and sleep problems.

A rapid drop in GH levels or an overt deficiency (a deficiency is characterized by IGF-1 readings below 90 µg/mL) can and should be treated, but a gradual decline over a period of years appears to be one of the body's ways of preventing cancer. Research now links elevated IGF-1 levels to increased risk for colon, pancreas, endometrial, breast and prostate cancers.

MY RECOMMENDATION

GH is a powerful hormone that should be used only by people who have been diagnosed with a deficiency. Even in these cases, GH replacement should be monitored by a physician. To gain the benefits of extra GH without the dangerous risks, there is a much more effective—and less costly—strategy. I recommend a combination of aerobic exercise (such as walking and cycling) and weight-lifting, each performed for 30 minutes three times a week. Sleep also is important for maintaining healthy GH levels. There are a variety of supplements that claim to boost GH levels, but no good data support their use. Save your money for the gym.

Dizziness

Salsa dancing was what Terri, a 52-year-old professor, missed most. "For weeks, I've felt dizzy on and off. I've had to skip salsa classes because dancing makes it much worse," she told me.

Terri was experiencing *vertigo*—a sensation that oneself and/or one's surroundings are in motion, although there is no actual movement. The feeling is described as spinning, whirling or tilting. In severe cases, people may lose their balance and fall, feel nauseated and/or vomit.

A portion of the inner ear called the *labyrinth,* which includes three loop-shaped semicircular canals, contains special cells, called *hair cells,* that detect motion and changes in body position. An injury or disease of the inner ear can cause hair cells to send false signals to the brain. When the false signals conflict with signals from the eyes and areas of the brain involved in balance, vertigo occurs.

With Terri, I looked for signs of conditions that can cause vertigo—including anemia, infections, low or high blood sugar, low or high blood pressure, slow or rapid heartbeat, multiple sclerosis, stroke, migraines, head injury and inner ear tumors. I double-checked her medications, because vertigo is a possible side effect of some blood pressure and pain drugs, antidepressants and antibiotics. An ocean voyage can trigger vertigo that persists even after going ashore. However, Terri had no signs or history of any of these factors.

I surmised that Terri had *benign paroxysmal positional vertigo* (BPPV), in which "ear rocks" (small crystals of calcium carbonate and protein) become dislodged from their proper position and float in the fluid of the inner ear. This debris can irritate nerve endings associated with balance and cause a spinning sensation when a person moves. Dizziness occurs intermittently and lasts a few seconds to a few minutes. BPPV symptoms often subside without treatment within six months—but while they persist, it is hard to engage in normal activities.

Maneuvers of the head and body (called Epley or Semont maneuvers) can help move the debris to a less irritating area of the inner ear, often alleviating vertigo within minutes. An otologist (ear doctor) can perform these maneuvers, which may need to be repeated several times before they are effective.

Since Terri's symptoms were relatively mild and occurred primarily when she danced, we decided to start with a safe homeopathic remedy called *Cocculus* (from the cockle plant). No one knows exactly how Cocculus works, but it has a long history of success in treating vertigo and motion sickness. I told Terri to take two pellets of a 30C potency a half hour before dance class and again afterward.

Terri was afraid she would feel embarrassed if she got dizzy while dancing—but to her delight, the Cocculus worked the first time. She continued to use it for eight weeks, then stopped. Her vertigo did not return—and she could once again twirl comfortably in the arms of her dance partner.

markers were significantly lower as well in the low-calorie group.

My view: Calorie restriction has been shown to slow aging and prolong life span in other mammals. This was the first human study to show a correlation between calorie restriction and an antiaging effect on heart function. Researchers theorize that chronic inflammation from a typical calorie-loaded Western diet, which is heavy in animal products and refined sugar but low in fruits and vegetables, causes damage to—and premature hardening of—heart muscle. More studies are needed. Keep in mind that the quality of your food choices is as important as calorie restriction. For best results, opt for fruits, vegetables, cold-water fish, lean poultry, whole grains and legumes, limited red meat—and watch your portion sizes.

Calorie-Restricted Diet And Aging

A calorie-restricted diet could slow aging of the heart, according to new research. Investigators looked at lab reports and Doppler imaging of 25 people who had been practicing calorie restriction for about six years. The people, ages 41 to 65, consumed an average of 1,400 to 2,000 calories a day. Their blood pressure, heart function and inflammatory blood markers, including *C-reactive protein*—a measure of inflammation in blood vessels and elsewhere in the body—were compared to those of 25 people of similar age and gender with an intake of 2,000 to 3,000 calories per day, the amount in a typical Western diet. Researchers found that diastolic function of the heart in the calorie-restricted group resembled diastolic function in people about 15 years younger. (*Diastolic,* the bottom number in a blood pressure reading, measures the pressure when the heart is at rest, in between beats.) There was little difference in *systolic function* (the top number in a blood pressure reading, which measures the pressure inside blood vessels when the heart beats). Blood pressure overall and inflammatory

No More Eyestrain

Anyone who spends extended time at a computer (an hour or more without a break) is vulnerable to blurred vision, red eyes, difficulty seeing long distances and headaches.

One of the first steps is to eliminate glare by tilting the screen away from light or getting an antiglare screen. These screens ($35 to $50) are sold at office-supply and computer-accessory stores. Face your monitor away from windows and other bright light sources, and place it so the middle of the screen is slightly below eye level (about 20°).

Take a five-minute break every 45 to 60 minutes to relax your eyes and body. Get up and walk around, and look away from bright light. Then sit in a relaxed position—for example, with your back straight and your hands on your knees, and take deep breaths.

The herbal extract bilberry (available at health-food stores and pharmacies) improves circulation to the eyes and reduces the redness and irritation that many people experience from computer use. Take 320 mg daily of a 25% *anthocyanoside* extract. For best results, take bilberry indefinitely.

Simple, but Effective— Schussler Cell Salts

There are more than a thousand homeopathic remedies. Each one has its own set of symptoms on which it is used. The Schussler cell salts are a simplified system that complements other homeopathic remedies. As you will see, they are easy for the public and homeopaths to use. What is more important, they work!

Have you ever taken a mineral like magnesium to help reduce or prevent muscle cramps, and find that it does not help?

You may not be getting the benefit from the magnesium at the cellular level, no matter how much you are taking. In a case like this, I find that taking the cell salt, or the homeopathic form of the deficient mineral, works quickly to alleviate the condition. The cell salt stimulates a biochemical change at the cellular level, which then gives the desired result.

Dosage: Cell salts are used like other homeopathic remedies—and as with other homeopathics, they come in pellet, tablet or liquid form. The most common potency available commercially is 6x.

Cell salts are best taken 10 to 20 minutes before or after you have any drink or meal. For an infant, you can crush a cell salt tablet and place it on the child's tongue. Or you can mix the tablet with an ounce of purified water and place a few drops in the child's mouth using a dropper or teaspoon. Children like the sweet taste of the pellets and tablets.

When you do take cell salts, however, you'll probably want to avoid strong odors, such as the fragrance of eucalyptus or essential oils.

For acute conditions, cell salts should be taken every 15 minutes or 2 hours, depending on the severity of the condition. For chronic conditions, cell salts are usually taken one to three times daily. Since they are of a low potency, they can be used on a long-term basis.

As described below, one type of cell salts—or a combination of them—can be taken to treat a particular symptom or condition. For example, mag phos helps to relieve muscle spasms. If a person is also experiencing nerve pain, then kali phos could be used as well. These different types of cell salts can either be taken at the same time or in alternating doses throughout the day.

There are also some formulas that combine all the cell salts together in one formula. These are commonly known as bioplasma. They may be used preventatively or to recover from various chronic illnesses.

What are the side effects?: Side effects are not an issue with cell salts. They either help or do nothing at all.

SELECTING THE APPROPRIATE CELL SALT

A list of various cell salts follows, with the conditions for which each is used.

●**Calcarea (pronounced kalk-ar-ee-uh) fluorica (calc fluor).** This cell salt is involved in the formation of connective tissue, making it important for the skin, ligaments and tendons. It is also found in bones. *I recommend it for the following conditions…*

- Abnormal spine curvature
- Brittle teeth and sore gums
- Hard nodules of the breast or other tissues
- Hemorrhoids
- Spine that "goes out" easily (including during pregnancy)
- Sprains and strains
- Varicose veins, weak ligaments, tendons and joints

●**Calcarea phosphorica (calc phos).** This is the main cell salt for bone health. Interestingly, calcium phosphate is an important enzyme required for bone formation. Calc phos helps in bone formation. *I recommend it for the following conditions…*

- Arthritis
- Fractures
- Growing pains
- Osteoporosis
- Teething

●**Calcarea sulphurica (calc sulph).** This cell salt is a wound- and skin-healer. (It is especially recommended when there is a yellow discharge from the skin.) *I recommend it for the following conditions…*

- Abscess
- Acne
- Boils

•Bronchitis

•Post-nasal drip

•Ferrum phosphoricum (ferrum phos). This cell salt is homeopathic iron phosphate. It is required for red blood cell formation and function. *I recommend it for...*

•Anemia treatment and prevention (iron deficiency)

•Bleeding (acute and chronic)

•Fever and infection

•Heavy menstruation

•Kali (pronounced collie) muriaticum (kali mur). This cell salt helps to dissolve mucus. *I recommend it for the following conditions...*

•Fluid in the ears

•Sore throat (with white mucus being produced)

•Kali phosphoricum (kali phos). This is the primary cell salt for nervous tissue, including the brain. *I recommend it for...*

•Anxiety and nervousness

•Depression

•Fatigue

•Nerve injury

•Poor memory and lack of concentration

•Kali sulphuricum (kali sulph). This is another remedy for skin and mucous membrane discharges (especially where there is a yellow discharge). *I recommend it for...*

•Bronchitis

•Eczema

•Psoriasis

•Magnesia phosphorica (mag phos). This is the primary cell salt for the muscles—both internal and external. It also has a tonic effect on the nervous system as well. *It can help with...*

•Anxiety and nervousness

•Hyperactivity

•Menstrual cramps

•Muscle spasms and cramps

•Seizures

•Stomach cramps

•Toothache

•Natrum muriaticum (nat mur). This cell salt regulates water balance within the cells and tissues. *I recommend it for the following conditions...*

•Cold sores

•Depression

•Dry skin

•Edema

•Grief

•Hayfever

•Skin rash from sun exposure

•Natrum phosphoricum (nat phos). This is the cell salt that is an acid-base balancer of the cells. *I recommend it for the following conditions...*

•Bladder infections

•Heartburn

•Muscle soreness

•Vaginitis

•Natrum sulphuricum (nat sulph). This remedy has a balancing effect on the fluids of the body. In addition, it tonifies the liver and digestive tract. *I recommend it for...*

•Asthma

•Head injury

•Hepatitis

•Newborn jaundice

•Swelling

•Silica. This cell salt is found in the connective tissue, skin, glands and bones. It acts as a tissue cleanser. *I recommend it for the following conditions...*

•Acne

•Asthma

•Boils

•Brittle hair and nails

•Sinusitis

The Buzz About Apis

Apis (pronounced *aye-pis*) is a remedy that is derived from the honeybee—the stinger as well as the whole bee. Think of the symptoms that a bee sting causes such as stinging, burning, swelling and itching. These are all the symptoms for which apis is beneficial. So a homeopathic doctor may recommend it for bee stings, allergic reactions including hives, arthritis, urinary-tract infections, kidney disease, herpes, sore throat and ovarian pain.

Apis is indicated when symptoms include a lack of thirst, a negative response to heat and a positive response to cold applications.

Recommendations for…

●**Allergic reactions.** Allergic reactions that cause hives or burning and stinging pains that move around the body can be improved quickly with apis. Apis also improves other symptoms of allergic reaction such as swelling of the throat and eyes. These could be allergic reactions to food or to drugs.

Note: Seek emergency medical treatment for allergic reactions, especially if you start to have trouble catching your breath.

●**Arthritis.** If you have swollen joints that burn or sting—and if your joints feel better after applying cold compresses—then the condition can probably be alleviated with apis.

●**Bee stings.** Apis quickly relieves the pain of a bee sting. This is proof of the homeopathic principle that "like cures like." Take it as soon as possible after getting stung to prevent swelling and other symptoms from getting severe. Apis is a remedy that should be in your home first-aid kit.

●**Herpes.** Apis is a common remedy for herpes infections. Herpes of the mouth—cold sores that sting and burn and that have a vesicle formation—improves quickly with apis. This also applies to the acute treatment of genital herpes.

●**Kidney disease.** Apis is used in acute kidney disease such as glomerulonephritis or nephritic syndrome where there is protein loss in the urine and edema of the body.

●**Meningitis.** Symptoms include a stiff neck, high fever and dilated pupils. Homeopathic apis is most effective in patients whose symptoms are made worse when heat is applied. This remedy can be used in conjunction with conventional treatment.

●**Ovarian pain.** Apis is specific for right-sided ovarian cysts where there is burning and stinging pain. It not only reduces the pain, but also stimulates dissolving of the cysts.

●**Shingles.** Apis is one of the primary homeopathic medicines for shingles, especially when there is stinging or burning. Apis helps to relieve the pain and heal the shingles.

●**Sore throat.** Apis is very effective for relieving a sore and swollen throat, especially when the sore throat has specific characteristics. Those characteristics include a burning pain (that feels better when you have a cold drink) and a bright red, swollen uvula (the flap of tissue in the middle of the mouth).

●**Toxemia in pregnancy.** Apis is a good remedy for toxemia in pregnancy where there is protein in the urine, high blood pressure and lots of body swelling.

●**Urinary-tract infections.** Urinary-tract infections can be helped by apis. This is particularly true for bladder infections that cause scalding pain during urination. If you have a right-sided kidney infection, it's another indication that this remedy will probably work well.

Dosage: For acute conditions such as a bee sting or allergic reaction, I recommend taking the homeopathic formulation with a 30C potency every 15 minutes for two doses. Then wait and see if the remedy is helping. The other option is to take one dose of a higher potency such as a 200C.

For skin rashes, sore throats and other conditions that are not so acute, I recommend taking a 6C, 12C, or 30C potency twice daily for three to five days, or as needed for continued improvement.

What are the side effects?: Side effects are not an issue with apis. It either helps or there is no effect at all. It is also safe to use for children.

Keeping Up the Pressure—Amazing Way to Reduce Stress

Many people are aware of acupuncture as a treatment to relieve pain. However, acupressure has been used long before acupuncture in China, Japan and India. Actually, it could be said that most every culture used acupressure to some degree. Simply, it was pushing on "tender" spots to relieve local pain and discomfort. Sometimes, it's what we do naturally—pressing on a sore, aching muscle, for instance. But practitioners in acupressure and acupuncture have identified less obvious, specific points of the body that can contribute to pain relief or healing.

Chinese medicine has relied on acupressure for over 4,000 years. Today, it remains a major treatment at Chinese hospitals. Its popularity has been growing steadily throughout the world.

CHANNELS OF ENERGY

The traditional Chinese system of medicine focuses on the concept that the life-giving energy called *Qi* (pronounced *chee*) circulates throughout the body in 12 main channels. Each channel represents a certain organ system—such as kidney, lung and large intestine. The points that connect to that system are located bilaterally—that is, on both sides of the body. These channels are all interconnected, so they link up to one another.

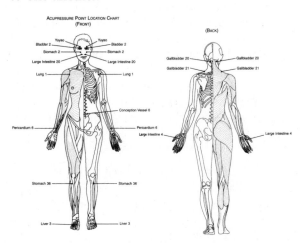

Along each of the channels, known as *meridians,* are specific acupressure points that can relieve local pain and inflammation, and also affect pain or tension in other areas of the body. Many of the points can be used to influence the function of internal organs. It is believed that when there is a blockage of Qi circulation in the channels, then disease or illness arises.

To prevent a disease from occurring, or to treat a disease, one must keep the Qi moving. One way to do this is to stimulate the acupressure points where a blockage is occurring. Usually these points are tender to the touch, indicating a blockage. Whether you relieve sore muscles

or an internal problem such as digestive upset depends on which points you press. Mental and emotional imbalances can also be helped with acupressure.

CHEMICAL REACTION?

It is not known exactly how acupressure relieves pain or improves the functioning of internal organs. One theory is that the brain releases certain chemicals that inhibit pain and stimulate the immune system. It is also thought that acupressure relaxes trigger points so muscle tension calms down.

Acupressure may improve blood and lymphatic circulation, as well as improve electrical flow along nerves and between cells. Much research is ongoing in this area, including studies funded by the prestigious National Institutes of Health. Acupressure does work and is a major reason why traditional Chinese medicine is one of the fastest growing medical fields.

While someone trained in acupressure can obtain the best results, there are many easy-to-locate points that you can apply pressure to yourself to alleviate discomfort or improve certain conditions.

ADMINISTERING AN ACUPRESSURE TREATMENT

Here are four easy steps to follow for self-treatment…

1. Make sure you are relaxed. The room should be free of noise. If possible, you should wear light clothing.

2. Locate the desired point to which you are going to apply pressure. Press on the point using your thumb or fingers. The pressure should be direct, yet not cause great discomfort. Some points may be very tender, indicating a blockage.

Start with very light pressure, see how you feel, and adjust the pressure accordingly. Press the acupressure point and hold for 10 to 15 seconds. This can be repeated 5 to 10 times to see if it helps relieve the symptoms.

Chronic conditions will need more treatments to see if the acupressure is working. Some people prefer rubbing or massaging the acupressure points; this is fine to do as well. As the same channel runs on both sides of the body, try to stimulate the points on both sides simultaneously.

For example, massaging Gallbladder 20 on both sides of the back of the head helps to relax tense neck muscles. Or, Stomach 36, located four finger widths below the kneecap and one finger width toward the outside of the leg (outside the shin bone on the muscle), can be stimulated simultaneously to improve digestive function.

3. Make sure to breathe while you stimulate the acupressure point. Slow, deep, relaxed breaths are best.

4. Relax in a quiet atmosphere after a treatment and drink a glass of water to help detoxify your body.

What are the side effects?: Acupressure is a very safe treatment. Temporary soreness of the acupressure point is common and normal. Acupressure should not be applied to open wounds or areas of extreme swelling or inflammation, such as varicose veins.

There are certain points that should not be stimulated on a pregnant woman because of the risk of miscarriage. It is important that pregnant women avoid the use of Gallbladder 21, Large Intestine 4 and Liver 3. Pregnant women should consult with a practitioner of acupressure before self-treating.

Recommendations from the Natural Physician for…

•Allergies.

•Large Intestine 4, located between the webbing of the thumb and index finger, relieves nasal symptoms and head congestion.

•Large Intestine 20, located on the lower, outer corner of each nostril, reduces sneezing and nasal symptoms.

•Anxiety.

•Pericardium 6, located two-and-one-half finger widths below the wrist crease in the middle of the forearm (palm side), helps relieve anxiety.

•Cold and flu.

•Large Intestine 4, located between the webbing of the thumb and index finger, relieves head congestion and sinus discomfort. Gently push on this spot. You want to work this acupressure point on both hands, so after you've treated your left hand, be sure to do the same to the right.

•Large Intestine 20, located on the lower, outer corner of each nostril, reduces sneezing and nasal symptoms.

•Cough.

• Lung 1, located in the front of the shoulder area, in the space below where the collarbone and shoulder meet, reduces cough.

•Constipation.

•Large Intestine 4, located between the webbing of the thumb and index finger, relieves constipation. Gently push on this spot on both hands.

•Eyestrain.

•Stomach 2, located one-half inch below the center of the lower eye ridge (you can feel an indentation), relieves burning, aching and dry eyes.

•Bladder 2, located on the inner edge of the eyebrows beside the bridge of the nose (you can feel an indentation), relieves red and painful eyes.

•Headache.

The following are all helpful. Choose the point or points that provide the most effective relief for you.

•Gallbladder 20, located below the base of the skull, in the space between the two vertical neck muscles.

•Large Intestine 4, located between the webbing of the thumb and index finger. Gently push on this spot on both hands.

•Liver 3, located on top of the foot in the hollow between the big toe and second toe.

•Yuyao, indentation in the middle of the eyebrow (directly straight up from pupil).

•Indigestion.

•Stomach 36, located four finger widths below the kneecap and one finger width toward the outside of the leg (outside of shin bone on the muscle), improves digestive function.

•Conception Vessel 6, located two finger widths below the navel, relieves abdominal pain, gas and other digestive problems.

•Muscle pain.

•Find the points that are most tender in the sore muscle and gently press on them and release, or massage these points.

•Nausea.

•Apply pressure on Pericardium 6, which is located two-and-one-half finger widths below the wrist crease in the middle of the inside of your forearm. This point works so well for nausea that special wrist bands can be bought that stimulate this point. They are used for any kind of nausea, including morning sickness and motion sickness.

•Conception Vessel 6, located two finger widths below the navel, relieves nausea and abdominal symptoms. It is also effective for motion sickness.

•**Neck pain.**

•Gallbladder 21, located on the highest point of the shoulder (*trapezius muscle*), relieves stiff neck and shoulder tension. Feel for a tender spot.

•Gallbladder 20, located below the base of the skull, in the space between the two vertical neck muscles, relieves stiff neck and neck pain.

•Large Intestine 4, located between the webbing of the thumb and index finger, reduces neck and head discomfort. Gently push on this spot on both hands.

•**Sinusitis.**

The following two points relieve sinus pain and promote drainage.

•Large Intestine 20, located on the lower, outer corner of each nostril.

•Large Intestine 4, located between the webbing of the thumb and index finger.

Waiter, More Water!

As we all probably learned in school, water is composed of two hydrogen molecules and one oxygen molecule. More than half of our total body weight is water, and a newborn is about three-quarters fluids and one-quarter solid, living human matter.

The brain, surprisingly, is the most concentrated reservoir. There, the concentration of water is almost 85 percent.

About two-thirds of the water in our systems comes from those glasses of fluids that we drink. The rest comes from food and from the leftover "disposables" of cellular metabolism.

Our bodies are really the middle of a streambed. While the water is coming in through various

pathways, it's exiting in the urine (60%), evaporating from skin (20%), hissing out through the respiratory tract (15%) and departing in stool (5%).

Water is involved in every single biochemical activity in the body and is required as a solvent for many processes. It is an important component of blood (plasma) and fluids inside and outside the cells. All the tissues of the body—including cartilage and skin—are unquenchable water drinkers. The medium of water is a traveling roadshow, where electrolytes move around, enabling the cells to perform their duty as they generate electrical activity. You need water for detoxification, because waste products course their way out of the body through the multitude of aqueducts—veins, arteries, glands and organs—that pump, feed and carry fluids from place to place. Throwing in some thermostatic responsibilities, water also provides a means for temperature regulation.

BODY LUBE

Humans have a thirst mechanism that is activated when our body is becoming low in reserves of water. Researchers have noted that there is often a long delay between the time when your body actually becomes dehydrated and the moment when you experience the sensation of thirst. In other words, by the time you feel thirsty, you're *already* somewhat dehydrated.

There are a number of symptoms of dehydration that you should be aware of. Thirst, naturally, is one—and any time your mouth feels dry or "sticky," you probably need fluids. Dark urine is another sign.

Many people are in a constant, low-grade state of dehydration. They won't faint, nor do they need to be hospitalized. But that low-grade dehydration can sap vitality and contribute to many of the symptoms I've noted.

Of course, there are situations that lead, almost automatically, to dehydration. If you're in a hot climate, exercising heavily and not drinking very much, your water reserves drop fast. But excessive sodium intake—eating a lot of salty foods, including heavily processed food products—will draw water out of the tissues. (I am always reminded of the effects of sodium a couple hours after eating sushi with soy sauce, or foods containing lots of sodium.)

THE DEHYDRATORS

If you drink a lot of beverages containing caffeine—coffee and soda, for instance—you're sure to have some dehydration unless you also drink lots of water. Alcoholic beverages also have a dehydrating effect.

Any medication that's described as a diuretic, or drugs that have diuretic side effects, will require you to compensate for water loss by getting more fluids every day.

Conditions I see that are related to insufficient water intake include headaches, dizziness, heart palpitations, high blood pressure, irritability, cloudy thinking, skin rashes, kidney pain and fatigue. Other physicians have noted even more conditions associated with dehydration, ranging from colitis and rheumatoid arthritis to obesity, asthma and allergies.

Of course, while I'm recommending that people drink sufficient water, I'm acutely aware that many are concerned with the quality of their drinking water. Thousands of people suffer from parasites and other infections related to contaminated water each year. Industrial pollutants and chemicals are traceable in many sources of drinking water. Even the chemicals used to purify water—such as chlorine—have in some cases been linked to cancers such as bladder cancer and, possibly, aggravating asthma. Heavy-metal contamination such as lead, mercury and aluminum are problems as well.

I advise people to invest in a high-quality filtration system or drink tested bottled water. I also recommend having your local water tested.

Dosage: Drink at least six to eight 8-ounce glasses of water daily. If you drink coffee, consume one 8-ounce glass of water for every cup of coffee you drink.

If the weather is hot, drink a glass or two before exercising, and have more than eight glasses during the day.

People on detoxification programs often need to increase their water intake to help flush toxins out of the body.

What are the side effects?: In rare cases, too much water consumption may place stress on your heart or kidneys. If you have kidney or heart disease, consult with your doctor before drinking larger-than-normal amounts of water.

You may feel bloated if you haven't been drinking very much water and then abruptly increase your water intake. The bloating comes from swallowing extra air—but it won't take long for your body to adjust to increased water intake.

Recommendations from the Natural Physician for…

• **Cloudy thinking.** I call this symptom "brain fog," and most people know instantly what I mean. The mind is not clear, and you find it hard to concentrate. I have seen these symptoms improved with increased water consumption.

• **Dizziness.** Unexplained dizziness may be related to dehydration. Water is required for normal blood pressure. When you're dehydrated, your circulation may be poor, which deprives cells of needed nutrients. Dizziness is one outcome.

• **Fatigue.** Unexplained fatigue can be a result of dehydration. Many people notice increased energy when they drink more water.

• **Headaches.** Patients with chronic, low-grade headaches are often dehydrated. It is often described as a fuzzy sensation in the head.

• **Heart palpitations.** Occasionally a patient reports a history of heart palpitations. These episodes may improve or cease completely when water intake increases.

• **High blood pressure.** You'd think that anyone consuming lots of water would be raising their own blood pressure, but the opposite is true. When you're dehydrated, your body tries to compensate by increasing blood pressure. So for anyone with high blood pressure (hypertension), it's important to increase water intake.

• **Irritability.** There are many reasons for irritability, of course, but if you think dehydration might be one possible cause, there's a quick way to find out—just start drinking a lot more water, and see if your mood improves.

• **Kidney pain.** A number of patients experience kidney pain when they are not drinking enough water. Any kind of kidney pain should be taken seriously. But while you should see the doctor and explain your symptoms, it's also advisable to increase your intake of water. It can't do any harm—and that just might turn out to be the explanation of the problem.

•**Skin rashes.** The skin is a major organ of detoxification. If you're not getting enough water in your system to aid detoxification, you can begin to develop skin rashes of many sorts. Increase water consumption, and you'll help expel some of the accumulated toxins in the body. This is the quickest "first aid" I can think of for treatment of skin rashes.

•**Weight gain and edema.** Your body will retain water if you are chronically dehydrated. This condition, called edema, contributes to weight gain as well. Thus, increased water consumption is an important therapy for helping these conditions.

The All-Purpose Remedy—Licorice Root

In my experience, licorice root is the most versatile of all the herbs. Native to both Asia and the Mediterranean, it has been used by practitioners of Ayurvedic and Chinese medicine for over 5,000 years.

In fact, close to 50 percent of all Chinese herbal formulas contain licorice root. The ancient Chinese texts say it can suppress coughs and moisten the lungs, relieve spasms, and soothe the digestive tract. It is also called a "harmonizing" herb. This means that it helps other herbs to work more effectively to reduce their toxicity when used in a formula.

Licorice also helps detoxify the liver, supports the adrenal glands (your body's major guardians against stress), balances the hormones and has powerful anti-inflammatory effects.

IMMUNITY BOOSTER

Licorice contains two substances, *glycyrrhizin* (pronounced *gle-sir-heh-zin*) and *glycyrrhetinic* (pronounced *gle-sir-heh-ti-nic*) acid, that have been shown in animal studies to increase the body's supply of one of nature's most powerful antiviral agents—*interferon*. Interferon helps to keep viruses from reproducing and stimulates the activity of other beneficial immune cells, as well. That's probably why licorice root is found in so many Western, Chinese, Japanese and Ayurvedic formulas for treating infectious disease.

Licorice root is highly regarded among European physicians as one of the top herbal medicines for combating viral hepatitis. They use the intravenous form for the treatment of both hepatitis B and C.

DELICIOUS DETOXIFIER

The Chinese have found through many centuries of using licorice that it reduces the toxicity of other herbs, so they add it to many of their remedies. For example, traditional Chinese herbal formulas containing Ma Huang (containing the chemical ephedrine, which helps open respiratory passageways but can also cause stimulant effects, such as fast heartbeat, sweating and anxiety), almost always contain licorice root, which helps to prevent these unwanted side effects.

Note: The Chinese species of licorice root is *Glycyrrhiza uralensis*. I find it works very similar in action to the kind used in North America—*Glycyrrhiza glabra*.

Dosage: For most conditions, I recommend taking licorice in tincture, capsule or tablet form. As a tincture, take 10 to 30 drops two to three times daily. As a capsule, take 1,000 to 3,000 mg daily.

DGL extract comes in tablet form. Chew one or two tablets (380 mg per tablet) 20 minutes before meals or take between meals.

What are the side effects?: High dosages of licorice root (3,000 mg daily of the powdered extract or more than 100 mg of the constituent glycyrrhizin) taken over many days can have effects similar to those associated with the hormone aldosterone. These include sodium and water retention, and potassium loss, which can lead to high blood pressure. We saw this problem occur when practitioners began recommending very high dosages of licorice root for adrenal burnout and chronic fatigue (which it can help).

Overall, I feel the risk of developing high blood pressure from using licorice is greatly exaggerated. Historically, herbalists have used this root in formulas for thousands of years. The trick is to use it in small amounts.

I do hear the occasional story of someone who feels that taking small amounts of licorice root has caused an increase in his or her blood pressure. This is possible for people who are very sensitive to licorice root or who have low levels of potassium. As a matter of fact, anyone concerned about high blood pressure should increase his or her intake of potassium-rich foods (bananas, orange juice, vegetables, etc.) and decrease the intake of sodium-containing foods (table salt, canned foods and restaurant foods). Using table-salt substitutes, which usually contain potassium, can help reduce sodium intake. Multivitamins also contain potassium.

Unless instructed to do so by a natural health-care practitioner, people who have kidney failure and hypokalemia (low potassium blood levels) should avoid using licorice root. Likewise, pregnant women and people with high blood pressure should use it with caution and under medical supervision. Whole licorice extract should not be combined with digitalis and diuretic medications. Taking only the DGL extract (for ulcers) eliminates most of the potential risk for high blood pressure.

Recommendations for…

•**Coughs.** Licorice is an excellent herb to use for coughs, both wet and dry. Licorice has a moistening and soothing effect for dry coughs. It also has a direct cough suppressant effect and is a common ingredient in throat lozenges.

•**Detoxification.** Licorice is one of the herbs to consider when undergoing a detoxification program. As I mentioned, it helps support the liver and should be considered along with herbs like milk thistle and dandelion root. It also works to heal a damaged digestive tract, which is key to long-term detoxification success.

•**Eczema and psoriasis.** Creams containing glycyrrhetinic acid are used to treat inflammatory skin conditions such as eczema and psoriasis. Its effect is similar to that of topical cortisone, and some studies have found it more effective. However, I do not recommend topical treatments (whether natural or pharmaceutical) as the main therapy for skin conditions, as they can simply mask a symptom without treating its underlying cause (e.g., food sensitivities, poor digestion, nutritional deficiencies). Topical treatments are fine, so long as you also address the internal imbalances that are creating the symptom.

•**Fatigue.** People who experience high levels of stress for long periods of time can suddenly find that their adrenal glands can no longer pro-

duce balanced levels of stress hormones, such as DHEA, pregnenolone and cortisol. As a result, fatigue, poor memory, blood-sugar problems, decreased resistance to illness and hormonal imbalance can occur.

Some doctors immediately recommend using hormone replacement, and in some cases this is necessary. However, it is worth trying a gentler approach, using supplements such as licorice root, especially to balance out cortisol levels. A typical adult dosage would be 1,000 to 2,000 mg of licorice root extract taken daily for two months or longer.

Other supplements that work synergistically to treat this condition include adrenal glandular, ginseng, pantothenic acid, vitamin C, beta carotene and zinc. In more serious cases, hormones such as DHEA, pregnenolone, and even cortisol may need to be used.

•**Hormone imbalance.** Licorice is one of the better hormone-balancing herbs. It appears to have a balancing effect between estrogen and progesterone, and reduces excess testosterone levels. It is commonly included in formulas for PMS and menopause.

•**Infections.** As mentioned earlier, licorice root is very good for the immune system. The soothing and anti-inflammatory effect of licorice makes it especially good for respiratory tract infections.

•**Inflammation.** Licorice has potent anti-inflammatory properties. Glycyrrhizin is an important constituent that improves the effects of cortisol in the body (powerful anti-inflammatory and anti-allergy effects), without the side effects seen with pharmaceutical anti-inflammatory agents such as prednisone. It also inhibits the formation of prostaglandins, which are substances in the body that cause inflammation.

•**Inflammatory bowel disease.** Licorice root is often included in formulas designed to heal conditions such as Crohn's disease and ulcerative colitis.

•**Mouth sores.** Mouth sores, also called aphthous ulcers, can be helped by licorice root. One study of 20 people found that a DGL mouthwash improved the symptoms of 15 of the participants by 50% to 75% within 1 day, and complete healing of the sores within 3 days.

97

.Ulcers. One of the most popular uses of licorice extract is for ulcers of the digestive tract. The recommended form is DGL. It has an interesting mechanism of action: It stimulates cell growth of the stomach and intestinal linings, increases the natural mucous lining of the stomach, increases blood flow to the damaged tissues and decreases muscle spasms.

In a single-blind study of 100 people with peptic ulcers, participants took either DGL (760 mg three times daily) or the medication Tagamet (cimetidine). Both groups showed equally significant healing of ulcers after 6 and 12 weeks, demonstrating that DGL is as effective as pharmaceutical medications for this condition. Another study of 874 people also demonstrated that DGL was as effective as antacids and the antiulcer drug cimetidine in persons with duodenal ulcers.

More important, DGL actually works to heal ulcerated tissues instead of simply suppressing stomach acid in the way antacids and drug medications do. Remember, with insufficient stomach acid, you cannot digest proteins, minerals and other nutrients very efficiently. Stomach acid also acts as a natural barrier that keeps bacteria, parasites and other microbes from penetrating the digestive tract.

The Benefits of Moving And Shaking—Exercise

I wrote this section after coming back from a 3-mile run. I felt great—and knew why. Every time anyone does exercise like this, there's a surge in endorphins and enkephalins—the body chemicals that make you feel good. I was highly motivated to discuss this major component of health and vitality.

Exercise is essentially some form of movement. This ranges from walking to jogging, from biking to playing tennis, to dancing and tai chi and all the other forms of movement you can think of.

Many people think of a gym when they hear the word *exercise*. For some people this brings up images of large muscular men or women grunting and groaning as they lift weights. They equate "exercise" with painful exertion.

My goal here is to get you motivated to exercise and then to select exercises that excite you. I also want you to realize the benefits of exercise and what it can do for you physically and mentally. In addition, I want to give you a sense of what kind of exercise you may want to be doing.

GETTING STARTED

The first step to a successful exercise program is to get motivated. Think of the health improvements you can get by exercising. Also, think how the quality of your life will improve when you lose weight, gain muscle and have an abundance of energy.

With more exercise, many areas of your life can improve, including relationships and work. Exercise is also an effective way to increase sex drive and libido naturally in men and women.

Next, think about what will happen if you don't exercise. See yourself as out of shape, having less energy and your body "falling apart." It's not a pleasant sight. Make up your mind right now that you will begin to figure out and implement an exercise program immediately. Feel good about it and get excited.

I think it's a mistake to select an exercise that you don't really like. For example, a friend invites you to go jogging, so you go, but you really have no interest in jogging. You would rather go swimming. If you pick an exercise that you don't have an interest in, you are not likely to stick with it. For an exercise program to be worthwhile, you have to stick with it over the long term. Studies show that if you abruptly stop exercising, you lose within a couple of weeks most of the benefits that you gained.

Besides motivation, compliance is everything when it comes to getting the benefits of exercise and sticking to an exercise program long term. By choosing one or two forms of exercise that you really enjoy, you increase your chances of sticking with it. Exercise should be something to which you look forward. It's something from which you can gain energy.

CHOOSING THE MIX

When choosing your exercise program, focus on aerobic work first. By this I mean walking, jogging, biking, swimming, tennis, dancing—any activity that keeps you constantly moving.

By contrast, there is also anaerobic exercise —such as weight lifting—but it's secondary. For example, weight lifting can improve muscular strength, muscle mass and bone density. It is also good for the heart and cardiovascular system. However, I recommend beginning with an aerobic exercise program, and then adding an anaerobic exercise like weight lifting.

A combination of cardiovascular training like walking or swimming (or many others) plus some form of resistance training like weights is best. This works all the systems of the body.

Don't feel you have to engage in vigorous physical activity to get the benefits of exercise. A study of more than 72,000 female nurses found that women who walk briskly five or more hours a week cut their risk of heart attack by 50 percent.

FREQUENCY AND LENGTH OF EXERCISE

The frequency and length of exercise depends on your current level of health. Your doctor and a fitness trainer can best determine this. In general, moderately healthy people should start with 10 to 15 minutes of aerobic exercise three times a week and work up from there.

Over time, the length of the exercise period can be increased to 30 to 45 minutes, and the frequency should be four to six times a week. If you experience muscle soreness, and it does not seem to be going away, then cut down the frequency and length of your exercise. If you're starting a weight-lifting program, be sure to work with a personal trainer.

If you want some guidance in starting an exercise program, I recommend *Weight Training for Dummies* by Liz Neporent, Suzanne Schlosberg and Shirley J. Archer, and *The Aerobics Program for Total Well-Being* by Kenneth H. Cooper.

What are the side effects?: Initially, muscle soreness will be the most common side effect as your body becomes accustomed to the exercise. This soreness will become less of a problem after the first three weeks. Proper form is required for weight lifting; otherwise, injuries can occur. In addition, proper warm-up and post-exercise stretching are important to prevent soreness and injuries.

Recommendations for...

•**Anxiety and depression.** Exercise reduces the effects of stress on the body and should be an important part of a treatment program for anyone with these conditions. It also stimulates the release of chemicals in the brain that are important for mood.

A study reported in the *Journal of Epidemiology* showed that those who participated in exercise, sports and physical activity experienced a decrease in depression, anxiety and malaise.

•**Arthritis.** The right kind of exercise can be helpful for the different forms of arthritis. For example, swimming is a good choice of exercise for someone with rheumatoid arthritis or osteoarthritis as it is gentle on the joints. Exercises performed improperly, such as running on a hard surface or using an improper weight-lifting technique, can aggravate arthritis.

•**Detoxification.** Regular exercise is helpful for anyone in a detoxification program. It promotes increased circulation and lymphatic drainage. It also causes sweating, and thus stimulates detoxification.

•**Diabetes.** Exercise increases insulin activity, reduces total cholesterol and triglycerides, and increases the good HDL cholesterol in those who have diabetes. It also stimulates blood flow that is more easily impeded in someone with this condition. However, anyone who has diabetes should be monitored by his or her doctor, and follow an exercise program under medical supervision.

•**Fatigue.** By expending energy, you can actually increase your energy and vitality level. This is the paradox of exercise, which works well to increase energy levels when done within the parameters of a person's exercise limits. On the other hand, over-exercise can lead to fatigue.

•**Heart disease.** It is a well-known fact that exercise reduces the risk of most cardiovascular diseases. Part of this effect comes from the lowering of cholesterol and triglycerides, and the increase in good HDL cholesterol. It also helps to reduce the effects of stress, another big risk factor for heart disease. Exercise also strengthens the heart muscle. However, anyone who has heart disease should be monitored by his or her doctor, and follow an exercise program under medical supervision.

•**Hot flashes.** Regular exercise has been shown to reduce the number of hot flashes that women experience during menopause.

•**Immunity.** Exercise done in moderation strengthens the immune system. For example, breast-cancer risk is reduced in women who exercise. But it's important to note that overtraining, as seen sometimes in marathon runners or triathletes, for example, can lead to suppression of the immune system. Again, balanced exercise is the key.

•**Osteoporosis.** It is undisputed that weight-bearing exercise stimulates the growth of bone cells and thus increases bone density. Actually, swimming and some other forms of less weight-bearing exercise have also proven to be effective. This is why exercise is so important to prevent and help treat osteoporosis.

•**PMS.** Regular exercise is quite helpful for women who consistently suffer from premenstrual syndrome.

•**Stress.** Exercise is one of the most effective techniques to alleviate the effects of stress on the body and mind.

SPECIAL REPORT #5:

Help or Hype?
The Truth About What Works
And What Doesn't

Help or Hype?
The Truth About
What Works and
What Doesn't

The Truth About Vitamin E

For more than 30 years, vitamin E has been one of the most widely used supplements. It's been touted as a key antioxidant, helping to prevent heart disease, certain cancers and other serious illnesses. But two years ago, vitamin E became quite controversial, because a few studies showed that it could be harmful. So it left many people wondering, *Is vitamin E safe? Is it effective? For what conditions? And what type of vitamin E should one use?*

Vitamin E is found naturally in wheat germ, nuts, seeds, whole grains, egg yolks and leafy, green vegetables. Animal products are a poor source of vitamin E. The recommended dietary allowance for vitamin E is 15 mg, or approximately 22 international units (IU), per day. Serious vitamin E deficiency is rare, although many Americans don't get enough of the vitamin. People on low-fat diets are susceptible to low vitamin E levels, because fat is needed for absorption of vitamin E. And people with the genetic condition cystic fibrosis have trouble absorbing vitamin E.

Vitamin E has been shown to be important as a supplement for people with specific diseases, such as Alzheimer's and diabetes, and those with a high susceptibility to certain conditions, such as bladder cancer and eye disease. Vitamin E prevents LDL "bad" cholesterol from becoming oxidized (damaged), thereby helping to guard against plaque formation in the arteries, known as atherosclerosis. Also, low vitamin E levels are associated with an increased risk of major depression, rheumatoid arthritis and preeclampsia (a condition during pregnancy characterized by high blood pressure and swelling of the hands and face).

Mark A. Stengler, ND, naturopathic physician in private practice, La Jolla, California...adjunct associate clinical professor at the National College of Natural Medicine, Portland, Oregon...author of many books, including *The Natural Physician's Healing Therapies* and coauthor of *Prescription for Natural Cures* (both from Bottom Line Books)...and author of the *Bottom Line/Natural Healing* newsletter.

103

CONTROVERSIAL STUDIES

Two recent, well-publicized studies have raised questions about vitamin E. The first was a meta-analysis (a study of other studies) led by researchers from the Johns Hopkins School of Medicine. The researchers reviewed 19 vitamin E studies that followed almost 136,000 patients. Most of these studies targeted populations at high risk for a chronic disease, usually coronary heart disease. Nine of the 19 studies focused on vitamin E alone, while the other 10 studies combined vitamin E with other vitamins or minerals. These studies ranged from 1.4 to 8.2 years in length. Vitamin E dosage varied from 16.5 IU to 2,000 IU per day, with a median dosage of 400 IU per day. The meta-analysis found that those taking 400 IU or more of vitamin E daily for at least one year were 10% more likely to die from all causes than those who took a smaller dose.

There are several problems with this analysis. First, researchers combined data that used both natural supplements (which provide the same type of vitamin E as that found in food) and synthetic forms of supplemental vitamin E. Previous research has shown that natural forms of vitamin E are better utilized by the body than cheaper, synthetic forms. The 1996 Cambridge Heart Antioxidant Study used only a natural form of vitamin E and found that a dose of at least 400 IU daily substantially reduced the rate of nonfatal heart attacks after one year of use.

The biggest criticism of the meta-analysis was that most of the studies included elderly people who had existing health problems such as cancer, Alzheimer's disease, heart disease and other potentially fatal illnesses. Even the authors of the research stated, "The generalizability of the findings to healthy adults is uncertain. Precise estimation of the threshold at which risk increases is difficult."

Another study, which was published in the March 16, 2005, issue of the *Journal of the American Medical Association,* focused on patients age 55 or older with vascular disease or diabetes. The study concluded that for people with vascular disease or diabetes, long-term supplementation with natural vitamin E does not prevent cancer or cardiovascular events and may increase risk for heart failure. This study provides no evidence that vitamin E is unsafe for people who are healthy.

POSITIVE FINDINGS

Many studies exist that demonstrate both the safety and effectiveness of vitamin E (in natural and synthetic forms). *A few examples…*

•**A Harvard study of more than 80,000 healthy,** female nurses ages 34 to 59 found a 41% reduction in the risk of heart disease in those who had taken daily vitamin E supplements of 100 IU or more for at least two years.

•**A study of almost 40,000 male health professionals** ages 40 to 75 found that those who took daily vitamin E supplements of at least 100 IU for more than two years experienced a 37% lower risk of heart disease.

•**A National Institute of Aging study focusing on 11,000 people between the ages of 67 and 105** found that those who used vitamins C and E supplements in various dosages had a 53% reduction in mortality from heart disease and a 42% reduction in death from all causes, compared with nonusers.

•**One study of moderate-severity Alzheimer's patients** conducted at Columbia University in New York City showed that a very high daily dose of vitamin E (2,000 IU) delayed the progression of Alzheimer's disease.

DIFFERENT TYPES

Vitamin E really refers to a family of compounds. There are more than 12 vitamin E compounds found in nature (currently eight forms are available in supplement form). There are two main groups of compounds—*tocopherols* (found in foods such as corn, soy and peanuts) and *tocotrienols* (found in rice, barley, rye and wheat). Many foods contain a blend of these two groups. Both have subgroups called *alpha, beta, gamma* and *delta.*

The most commonly used natural supplement form is *alpha-tocopherol,* and most studies have researched this form. But if you take just alpha-tocopherol you can reduce blood levels of gamma- and delta-tocopherols, which is not a good thing. Epidemiological (population) studies indicate that higher blood gamma-tocopherol levels correspond to the reduction of prostate cancer and coronary heart disease. Also, delta- and gamma-tocotrienols reduce the liver's production of cholesterol. One of the positive aspects of the negative vitamin E studies I mentioned earlier is that they have pushed researchers to look deeper into what vitamin E supplements should really contain.

I spoke with Barrie Tan, PhD, president of American River Nutrition, Inc., and adjunct professor of food science at the University of Massachusetts, Amherst, who is a specialist in the production and supplementation of vitamin E. He explains that 70% of (dietary) vitamin E consumed by North Americans is the gamma-tocopherol form due to the abundance of soy and corn in our diets. He believes that vitamin E supplements used for disease prevention should be a blend of both tocopherols and tocotrienols. I agree with this view, because these forms are more similar to what we find in food.

One example of a full-spectrum vitamin E product that has a good ratio of tocopherols and tocotrienols is Now Foods' Tru-E BioComplex. To find a health-food store that sells this product, call 888-669-3663 or go to *www.nowfoods. com*. A good dosage for anyone, healthy or not, is 200 IU daily. Consult with your doctor before using dosages above 400 IU, especially if you are taking a blood-thinning medication, such as *warfarin* (Coumadin)—vitamin E can have a blood-thinning effect.

Kombucha Tea

Kombucha tea was heavily promoted 15 years ago as a "natural mushroom" drink that increases energy, boosts immunity, alleviates joint pain and improves digestion. It also treats diabetes, cancer and many other maladies.

Kombucha is actually not a mushroom-derived tea but rather a mixture of different yeasts and bacteria that are fermented with sugar to produce a tea. When it was first introduced, people bought the yeast and bacteria starter-culture kits and combined them with black or green tea and sugar and let the mixture ferment for several days. The resulting "fermented tea" was supposed to promote healing. The product was just intriguing enough that a lot of people tried it, but its popularity died down after a few years.

Today, kombucha is re-emerging as a health tonic in the homemade tea and retail beverage market. I have been told that one national chain of health-food stores is having trouble keeping the product on its shelves.

Eye-popping ads on the Internet claim that kombucha is effective against AIDS, cancer, diabetes, hair loss, high blood pressure and several other conditions. When you see a long list of curative properties for any product, it should raise a red flag. Products that have no science or practical logic behind them tend to use smoke screens for promotion. A classic tactic is to describe a mysterious, beneficial product that is specifically used as a common cure in a foreign land.

Kombucha is claimed to have been a "fountain of youth" tea in China for thousands of years. It is said to have been used for sacred rites in China and the folklore to have been passed down through generations of family and friends. I have several friends who grew up in China and are now doctors, and they know nothing of this traditional use.

SAFETY CONCERNS

I am concerned about the safety of home-brewed kombucha tea. When the tea is made at home, contamination with potentially dangerous molds or bacteria is possible. Occasionally, there are reports of the home-brewed variety containing *Aspergillus,* a type of fungus that can produce harmful toxins that can cause diarrhea and vomiting if ingested. The Centers for Disease Control and Prevention (CDC) evaluated the tea when people reported getting sick after drinking it. The CDC also advises against home-brewed kombucha tea. Bottled kombucha tea from a health-food store is more likely to have been tested for contaminants. According to the Food and Drug Administration (FDA), it "has evaluated the practices of the commercial producers of [kombucha] and has found no pathogenic organisms or hygiene violations."

THEORETICAL BENEFITS

I am not aware of any scientific studies that have investigated the medicinal qualities of kombucha. If there is a benefit to this product, it may come from the acetic acid it contains. Acetic acid, also found in vinegar, appears to have a blood sugar–balancing effect and may possibly work as a mild weight-loss aid. Of course, one could more easily use apple cider vinegar (one tablespoon diluted with an equal amount of water and taken at the beginning of each meal) for the same purpose. It is safer and has been extensively studied.

My view: I do not recommend drinking kombucha tea for any health benefits. If you want to try the tea, buy the commercial variety, although I have no experience with any of the available brands. I advise against brewing kombucha at home, especially for consumption by the elderly, immune-compromised people or children.

Organic Foods... Worth the Cost?

"**O**rganic" is the buzzword these days, not just in natural-food stores but even in conventional supermarkets. But what does the term mean? Are organic foods really important for your health?

Under USDA guidelines, organic means the food hasn't been contaminated with man-made chemicals. Organic crops also are produced by farmers whose growing methods conserve soil and water. This helps ensure sustainable and nutritious produce for future generations.

Foods from all major food groups are available in organic form. Organic meat, poultry, eggs and dairy products come from animals that have not been given antibiotics or growth hormones. Animal feed also must be organic. Organic fruits, vegetables and grains come from fields that have been free of synthetic fertilizers and pesticides for at least three years. The foods must be grown without treated sewage sludge, which is commonly used as fertilizer. Organic farmers use animal manure, composted plant material, etc.

Organic farmers also avoid ionizing radiation—the process of applying radiation to raw meat, poultry and produce. In meats, the process kills pathogenic bacteria and other microorganisms. In produce, it kills spoilage-causing

bacteria and lengthens shelf life. Instead of radiation, organic farmers follow strict hygiene and sanitation practices and climate control—such as that provided by refrigeration.

There are many classifications for organic foods, and the rules can be tricky. A food that is 100% organic can be labeled "USDA organic" or "100% organic." Foods with mixed ingredients that are at least 95% organic also can use this seal. Foods in which at least 70% of the ingredients are organic (excluding salt and water) can highlight organic ingredients on the front of the package. If a product contains less than 70% organic ingredients, they may be called out on the side of the box, but the term "organic" can't appear on the front.

Organic produce prices vary but usually are only slightly higher than those of conventional fruits and vegetables. Organic dairy products are typically 15% to 20% more expensive than conventional dairy products, and organic meats and poultry cost two to three times as much as their traditional counterparts.

A RICHER SOURCE OF MINERALS

One study published in the *Journal of Applied Nutrition* compared the amount of healthful minerals and toxic metals in organically and conventionally grown produce—apples, potatoes, pears and sweet corn—as well as wheat. Over a two-year period, average levels of essential minerals were much higher in organic foods than in conventional foods. In addition, organic foods, on average, contained 25% less mercury and 29% less lead than conventional foods—both metals are toxic to the nervous and immune systems.

Pesticides, which are known hormone disrupters and suspected toxins to the nervous and immune systems, are a concern of mine. More than 1 billion pounds of pesticides and herbicides are sprayed on US crops each year. I believe that pesticides may contribute to the development of cancers of the breast, bone marrow and prostate.

Research has shown that people who live in agricultural areas where pesticides are used have an increased mortality rate from Parkinson's disease, a degenerative disorder of the nervous system. I am especially concerned about children who consume pesticides and other toxins in food. Of course, the absence of hormones and antibiotics in organic dairy and meat makes these foods more healthful than nonorganic varieties.

While organic foods cost more, they are worth the extra expense. However, it's still better for children and adults to eat nonorganic produce than to avoid it altogether.

Best: Incorporate organic foods—particularly dairy and produce—into your diet as much as possible.

as digestive upset. Even if you have only mild pain, these supplements can help prevent cartilage breakdown so that the problem does not worsen. For high-quality formulas, use brands sold at health-food stores.

Caution: Glucosamine and chondroitin may increase insulin resistance, so people with diabetes should monitor blood sugar levels carefully. The combination supplement should not be used by people with shellfish allergies.

Arthritis Supplements Do Help

Many patients have asked me about the well-publicized Glucosamine/Chondroitin Arthritis Intervention Trial. This six-month, multicenter clinical trial tested glucosamine and chondroitin as a treatment for knee osteoarthritis. In the study, 1,583 participants (average age 59) with knee osteoarthritis pain were randomly assigned to one of five treatment groups for 24 weeks: Glucosamine alone (1,500 mg per day)...chondroitin alone (1,200 mg)...glucosamine and chondroitin (1,500 mg and 1,200 mg, respectively)...200 mg of the prescription anti-inflammatory drug *celecoxib* (Celebrex)...or a placebo.

Researchers concluded that "glucosamine and chondroitin sulfate alone or in combination did not reduce pain effectively in the overall group of patients with osteoarthritis of the knee." As a result, many media outlets reported that glucosamine and chondroitin were ineffective for the treatment of osteoarthritis. While the combination wasn't effective for mild sufferers in the study, it was more effective than Celebrex for participants with moderate to severe osteoarthritis pain of the knees. Yet most of the mainstream media did not report this finding. Interestingly, for the group of patients with moderate to severe pain, Celebrex was only mildly more effective than the placebo.

My view: If you are being helped by these supplements, keep taking them. It's also worthwhile to try them before taking Celebrex or a similar drug, since glucosamine and chondroitin have a much lower risk of side effects, such

Garlic—Good...or Good for Nothing?

Does garlic stink at lowering cholesterol, as a recent study from Stanford University concluded? Or should we believe in previous evidence of its heart-healthy benefits? Let's look at the facts.

The Stanford study, published in *Archives of Internal Medicine,* involved 192 adults with moderately elevated LDL "bad" cholesterol levels. Participants were randomly divided into four groups. Six days a week for six months, participants consumed either raw garlic (4 g) ...a powdered garlic supplement (1,400 mg)... aged garlic extract (AGE, 1,800 mg)...or a placebo. Participants' blood cholesterol levels were measured monthly.

Researchers' conclusion: None of the garlic forms used in the study "had statistically or clinically significant effects on LDL or other plasma lipid (blood fat) concentrations."

At first glance, this study seems to refute all claims of garlic's cardiovascular benefits—but digging deeper reveals its flaws. While the participants' baseline LDL range varied widely— from 130 milligrams per deciliter (mg/dL) to 190 mg/dL—their average baseline level was just 140 mg/dL. Since the optimal LDL level is anything below 130 mg/dL, this means that most participants' LDL was only mildly elevated to begin with—which makes it difficult to achieve a measurable therapeutic response.

Earlier studies published in various medical journals demonstrate that garlic in supplement form does reduce LDL, total cholesterol and triglycerides (blood fats). The most well-studied form is AGE (sold in health-food stores), used in more than 350 studies. Results show that AGE can reduce LDL cholesterol by up to 12%... total cholesterol by up to 31%...and triglycerides by up to 19%. I see no reason to disregard numerous positive studies in favor of the small Stanford study.

Furthermore, while it is beneficial to reduce LDL, it is even more important to prevent LDL *oxidation* (the interaction between oxygen molecules and LDL). LDL oxidation occurs when negatively charged molecules damage LDL, inducing an immune response that triggers the formation of plaque in the arteries. AGE does protect against LDL oxidation. Furthermore, AGE thins the blood...lowers blood pressure...and lowers blood levels of *homocysteine*—an amino acid that, when elevated, raises the risk of stroke, heart disease and vascular disease.

ADVANTAGE: AGED EXTRACT

Fresh garlic is not the best choice for treating elevated cholesterol levels. As soon as garlic is heated, many healthful components are destroyed—though some may be preserved by crushing garlic, then waiting 10 minutes before cooking it. Numerous garlic products are standardized to their content of allicin (a sulfur compound)—yet this is meaningless because *allicin* breaks down quickly. However, the aging of garlic (soaking sliced garlic in water or alcohol for up to two years) produces *S-allylcysteine*. This substance inhibits production of LDL by the liver, an effect similar to that of cholesterol-lowering statin drugs—but without the drugs' dangerous side effects, such as gastrointestinal problems, muscle damage and liver failure.

Bottom line: Garlic in the form of AGE has many cardiovascular benefits. People who take a blood thinner, such as *warfarin* (Coumadin), or the anticoagulant *ticlopidine* (Ticlid), should check with their doctors before taking AGE. Otherwise, I recommend twice-daily doses of 4 milliliters (ml) to 6 ml of liquid AGE, or 400 mg to 600 mg in tablet or capsule form. And don't worry about bad breath—most AGE products are odorless.

Hype About the "Blood Type" Diet

Does blood type hold the key to identifying an individual's ideal diet? In his best-selling book, *Eat Right for Your Type* (Putnam), naturopathic doctor Peter J. D'Adamo says that the different blood types—A, B, AB and O—respond differently to various foods, so a person should follow a diet compatible with his/her blood type.

Blood type depends on the presence of certain *antigens* (molecules that stimulate an immune response) on the surface of red blood cells. Antigens detect bacteria, viruses and parasites, then activate the immune system to form antibodies to combat the intruders. Type A antigens react to different types of intruders than type B antigens do. This is why blood transfusions must be done with the right blood type—because type A antigens form antibodies to type B blood, and vice versa. Type AB antigens react to both types of intruders, while type O contains no blood-type antigens.

Dr. D'Adamo says that blood-type antigens also react to different foods.

His assertions: Foods contain proteins called *lectins* that interact with incompatible antigens. This causes red blood cells to clump and leads to inflammation, which impairs various body systems. Dr. D'Adamo tested many food lectins, combining them with different types of blood and examining them under a microscope to see if clumping occurred. These observations form the basis for his dietary recommendations. *In summary, people with...*

• **Type A blood** should focus on fruits, vegetables and grains, plus plant proteins such as soy...limit fats and dairy...and avoid meat, fish and poultry.

• **Type B blood** can handle a varied diet of vegetables...various meats (but not chicken or pork)...some fish (not shellfish)...and dairy.

• **Type AB blood** should emphasize vegetables...lamb and turkey (not beef, chicken or pork)...certain fish (not shellfish, sea bass or halibut)...some dairy (not whole milk or ice cream)...and some grains (not buckwheat or barley).

• **Type O blood** should eat vegetables, meat and fish…limit grains (especially wheat) and legumes…and avoid dairy and eggs.

One criticism I have—this diet oversimplifies blood-typing markers. There are nearly two dozen different blood-group markers (RH factor is one example). If antigens react adversely with certain foods, so might these other markers—but the blood-type diet does not account for these. Also, research on interactions between lectins and red blood cells has been done mostly in the lab, yet test-tube reactions may not mirror what happens in the body. And most food lectins are destroyed by cooking or digestion and so are not absorbed into the bloodstream—which means lectins do not come in direct contact with antigens and thus cannot interact adversely.

I surmise that people who benefit from a blood-type diet do so because these regimens limit simple sugars, dairy and red meat, and encourage vegetables and herbs—healthful practices no matter what a person's blood type.

Using myself as an informal subject, I analyzed Dr. D'Adamo's advice based on my type A blood.

Findings: His advice to avoid dairy and red meat is on target, because these foods cause me digestive problems—yet so does soy, a food that's encouraged. Dr. D'Adamo also says that people with type A blood can handle wheat and other grains, but I get joint pain and gas from grains with *gluten* (a sticky protein).

Trap: Food sensitivities can develop over time because of a wide variety of influences, not just blood type.

Bottom line: If you are curious about the blood-type diet, there's no harm in trying it for a month. But in general, I advise sticking with a balanced diet that emphasizes vegetables, fruits, seeds and herbs…provides protein from eggs, soy, nuts, legumes and, if desired, fish and poultry…and includes a variety of whole grains, especially gluten-free. If you want to avoid foods to which your body may be uniquely sensitive, consult a holistic doctor for food allergy testing.

Does Red Wine Protect the Heart?

You might have read the headlines in recent years—moderate consumption of alcohol, especially red wine, decreases the risk of cardiovascular disease. Before you assume that's reason enough to consume alcohol on a regular basis, let's look at this issue more closely.

It is true that alcohol consumption provides some cardiovascular protection. For example, when researchers combined data from 51 epidemiological studies, they found that the risk of heart disease decreased by about 20% when one to two alcoholic drinks were consumed per day. (One drink of alcohol is equivalent to 1.5 ounces of liquor, 5 ounces of wine or 12 ounces of beer.) The people who seemed to benefit most from light drinking (about 1.2 drinks a day) to moderate drinking (2.2 drinks daily) were middle-aged men and women.

Red wine has additional benefits over other alcoholic beverages, studies suggest. That's because several chemicals in red wine may protect the heart, including *resveratrol,* a polyphenol (plant pigment) with antioxidant effects. (White wine has smaller amounts of resveratrol.)

The natural compounds in red wine seem to prevent buildup of plaque in the arteries by reducing inflammation and promoting good tone in blood vessel walls. The compounds also play a role in preventing blood clots, which can obstruct blood flow and cause a heart attack or stroke. Alcoholic beverages of any type increase HDL "good" cholesterol, which removes LDL "bad" cholesterol from circulation, thereby minimizing plaque formation.

Despite these positive effects, I don't recommend that people rely on wine or any alcoholic beverages for heart disease prevention. If you do not drink alcohol on a regular basis, don't start. One of the obvious risks of regular alcohol consumption is alcoholism, a very serious and common disease in our country. *Other reasons not to drink alcohol…*

• **Cancer risk.** According to the American Cancer Society, men who have two alcoholic drinks a day and women who have one alcoholic drink a day increase their risk of certain cancers—of the esophagus, pharynx, mouth, liver, breast and colon. If you enjoy drinking each day, limit consumption to half a drink for women and one drink for men so as not to increase cancer risk.

• **Heart risk.** Paradoxically, the same amount of alcohol that has been shown to have a heart-protective effect—two drinks daily for men and one for women—also has been shown to raise triglyceride levels. High levels of these fats increase heart disease risk. Excessive drinking also raises the risk of high blood pressure, heart failure and stroke.

• **Obesity risk.** Alcohol contains simple carbohydrates. Consuming large amounts of simple carbs increases the risk of obesity and diabetes.

• **Fetal risk.** Mothers who drink alcohol during pregnancy predispose their babies to birth defects.

You can dramatically reduce your risk of heart disease without negative effects by not smoking, avoiding secondhand smoke, exercising regularly and consuming a Mediterranean-style diet. This diet is rich in fruits and vegetables, whole grains, nuts, seeds, legumes and olive oil—and has low to moderate amounts of dairy, fish and poultry and little red meat. You also might take fish oil with a combined EPA and DHA total of 500 mg daily to get heart-healthy essential fatty acids.

Also drink purple grape juice. It makes arteries more flexible and reduces the susceptibility of LDL cholesterol to cause damage in patients with coronary artery disease. Purple grape juice has potent antioxidant activity and, like red wine, contains resveratrol. It is high in simple sugars, so drink only six ounces daily—with a meal to slow sugar absorption. If you have diabetes, have no more than four ounces daily with a meal.

Harmful Heartburn Drugs

First the bad news: Popping a pill to alleviate heartburn can raise your risk for breaking a bone, getting an ulcer and perhaps even developing cancer. Since heartburn affects more than 60 million Americans at least once a month, the potential for harm is huge.

Heartburn (which has nothing to do with the heart) is not a disease, but a symptom—a burning sensation behind the breastbone. Most people have occasional heartburn (also called indigestion), usually brought on by a large or spicy meal.

Chronic heartburn usually signals *gastro-esophageal reflux disease* (GERD). Basically a mechanical malfunction, GERD occurs when the valve between the stomach and esophagus, called the lower esophageal sphincter (LES), fails to close properly, permitting stomach acid to back up. The esophagus doesn't have the stomach's strong protective lining, so acid damages esophageal tissues and causes pain.

GERD symptoms include persistent heartburn, acid regurgitation, chest pain, dry cough, bad breath and hoarseness in the morning. Untreated, GERD can scar the esophagus, making it hard to swallow…and may damage esophageal cell DNA, raising the risk of esophageal cancer.

Now for the good news: Natural treatments can safely heal GERD. Get the facts here—then work with your doctor to discontinue dangerous drugs as you incorporate natural therapies.

BANISH THE BURN, WEAKEN THE BONE?

Each year, GERD patients in the US are given about 100 million prescriptions for *proton pump inhibitors* (PPIs), which suppress the stomach's production of *hydrochloric acid*. PPIs include *rabeprazole* (Aciphex), *esomeprazole* (Nexium), *lansoprazole* (Prevacid), *omeprazole* (Prilosec) and *pantoprazole* (Protonix).

The *Journal of the American Medical Association* published an analysis of 16 years of medical records from 13,556 patients with hip fractures and 135,386 patients without fractures (all over age 50).

Conclusions: Patients who took PPIs at average doses for more than a year had a 44% increased risk of breaking a hip. Those who took higher-than-average doses more than doubled their risk of hip fracture.

Ironically, PPIs are often prescribed when GERD develops as a side effect of the osteoporosis drug *alendronate* (Fosamax). In other words, patients with brittle bones are given a drug to improve bone density…but the drug causes reflux, so patients are then given PPIs, which make bones even weaker!

Other GERD drugs that impede acid production include *histamine-2 receptor antagonists* (H2 blockers). Over-the-counter (OTC) H2 blockers include *cimetidine* (Tagamet HB), *famotidine* (Pepcid AC) and *ranitidine* (Zantac 75)—each of which also comes in prescription strengths. OTC *antacids,* which neutralize acids, have a similar effect. Antacids include *Alka-Seltzer, Maalox, Mylanta, Pepto-Bismol, Rolaids* and *Tums.*

What is the connection between acid-suppressing drugs and fractures? Hydrochloric acid promotes absorption of calcium and other minerals necessary for proper bone formation. When stomach acid is suppressed, the body cannot effectively absorb minerals—setting the stage for osteoporosis.

MORE REFLUX DRUG DANGERS

Stomach acid helps to break down protein into *amino acids,* which the body uses for tissue healing and immune response. When stomach acid is suppressed, protein is not properly digested. The resulting amino acids that are absorbed can trigger an *autoimmune reaction* (in which the immune system attacks the body's own tissues), causing pain and swelling of muscles, joints and digestive organs.

Heartburn drugs can decrease absorption of other drugs, too. These include some antibiotics, antifungals and the heart medication *digoxin* (Lanoxin).

When acid is low, *Helicobacter pylori*—a bacterium that causes stomach ulcers and increases the risk of stomach cancer—can flourish. So can fungi and bacteria that target the intestines, leading to bloating, diarrhea, constipation, gas and itchy rectum.

Paradoxically, drugs that reduce stomach acid can actually *increase* heartburn. When acid does not fully break down foods, the body may develop food sensitivities that further irritate the LES and stomach.

My view: GERD medications shouldn't be used—especially for more than a few weeks—unless natural treatments have been tried for four to six weeks and failed to alleviate heartburn and other symptoms.

ANTI-INDIGESTION DIET

Recently, a report in *Archives of Internal Medicine* reviewed 16 studies on the effects of changes in diet on heartburn symptoms. The report concluded that dietary restrictions did not help.

I adamantly disagree. The studies reviewed looked only at whether a particular food increased acidity in the stomach or decreased pressure exerted by the LES—but not at the real-world issue of whether avoiding that food alleviated symptoms. As hundreds of my patients can attest, heartburn may disappear with appropriate dietary changes. Avoid carbonated beverages, alcohol, coffee, nonherbal tea, cow's milk, citrus, chocolate, peppermint and spicy foods. If symptoms improve, reintroduce these foods one at a time to see which specific ones trigger your heartburn—and then avoid those foods in the future. If problems persist, a holistic doctor can test your sensitivity to different foods (using blood tests and other methods) to identify the culprits.

TRUSTED TRIO OF SAFE SOOTHERS

For further relief, I recommend the three natural GERD-combating supplements *par excellence.* All are sold at health-food stores and are safe for everyone (but not recommended for pregnant women).

Start with *aloe vera,* an anti-inflammatory plant that soothes the digestive tract lining. Three times daily, 20 minutes before meals, swallow 600 mg in capsule form…or four tablespoons of extract…or two teaspoons in powder form, mixed in water.

If heartburn persists after one week, add the homeopathic remedy *Nux vomica* to your regimen. Though no formal studies have been done, I believe that it strengthens the nerve impulses to the LES and helps it to close properly. Take two tablets of 30C potency twice daily until symptoms are gone. Thereafter, use as needed for occasional symptoms.

If symptoms remain after three weeks, also take *deglycyrrhizinated licorice root* (DGL). This stimulates the protective mucus of the stomach, soothing the LES and esophagus. Chew two 400-mg tablets three times daily, 20 minutes before meals.

Helpful: If heartburn makes it hard to sleep, avoid eating within two hours of bedtime. Also, raise the head of your bed six inches by placing wooden blocks beneath the bed frame's head two legs. Gravity helps keep stomach acid down, so heartburn is less likely to keep you up.

Help for Hiatal Hernias

Heartburn can result from a *hiatal hernia*—in which part of the stomach protrudes above the diaphragm (the muscle wall that separates the heart and lungs from the abdominal organs). This increases pressure on the lower esophageal sphincter (LES). It also irritates the *vagus nerve* (which carries messages from the brain to the digestive organs), reducing stomach acid production and stomach motility (movement) and delaying the passage of food into the intestines.

Solution: If an X-ray confirms the diagnosis, a chiropractor or holistic doctor can perform a gentle maneuver that moves the stomach downward, taking pressure off the LES and vagus nerve. Properly done, this maneuver is safe for everyone, except pregnant women. I teach patients' family members how to do this technique at home—but to prevent injury, do not try it without instruction from a professional.

With the patient lying face-up, I place my hands on the upper abdomen (over the stomach), then press firmly inward and downward for five seconds. Symptom relief, which can last for days or weeks, is usually immediate—and always welcome.

Whole-Food Multivitamins vs. Synthetic Supplements

Most nutritional supplements are synthesized—and thousands of studies show that they effectively prevent and treat disease. That said, it is best to get vitamins and minerals in the most natural form possible—from foods. Yet diet alone generally does not satisfy all our nutritional needs.

Whole-food supplements—foods that have been dehydrated, concentrated and powdered, then compressed into tablets or capsules, or sold as powders to be stirred into beverages—are an excellent way to help us meet those needs. Whole-food supplements may provide higher levels of certain phytonutrients (healthful plant chemicals) than synthetic ones do, and certain nutrients (such as vitamin E) are better absorbed in their natural form.

Some multivitamins that purport to contain whole foods offer only miniscule amounts, so select brands that contain therapeutic quantities. I like Nature's Way Alive! Whole Food Energizer Multi-Vitamin (800-962-8873, *www.naturesway. com*)…and New Chapter Every Man and Every Woman Multivitamins (800-543-7279, *www.new chapter.com*).

Airborne—Does It Really Fight Colds?

You probably know at least one person who never travels without Airborne, a dietary supplement introduced in the late 1990s. Since settling a recent lawsuit for false advertising, Airborne now promotes its product as an "immunity booster" rather than a preventive.

Company founder Victoria Knight-McDowell, a former elementary school teacher, had suffered from repeated colds in class and after traveling on airplanes. As the story goes, she worked with an herbalist from the University of California–Davis, as well as a nutritionist and a food scientist, to formulate her cold-fighting formula.

Airborne is a multinutrient tablet consisting of seven herbs, vitamin C and other antioxidants, electrolytes and amino acids. It has an effervescent delivery system—you drop one tablet in eight ounces of water, and it becomes a fizzy drink. Many of my patients think Airborne works well in treating the common cold.

Airborne's manufacturer has completed an unpublished study demonstrating the product's efficacy. To Airborne's credit, the trial was performed by an independent company that monitors clinical trials. This was a double-blind, placebo-controlled, randomized, multicenter study that compared adults with newly developed upper-respiratory tract infections (common colds) to people with common colds taking a placebo. The dose was one 1,000-mg Airborne tablet six times daily for five days. (That's higher than the recommended dose on the label—1,000 mg every three waking hours, as necessary.) Of the 48 participants who received Airborne, 48% reported noticeable relief from cold symptoms. Only 9% of the placebo group reported a similar level of relief.

I can see why people report benefits from this cold-fighting formula. *It provides many helpful ingredients...*

•**Vitamin C.** Airborne contains 1,000 mg of vitamin C per tablet. The debate about using vitamin C to treat the common cold rages on. However, several study reviews have found that it can significantly reduce the duration of colds and severity of symptoms. Although the dosage in the Airborne study was one 1,000-mg tablet six times per day, you can get a therapeutic effect—relief or prevention of cold symptoms—by taking 3,000 mg of Airborne daily. The most common side effect is loose stools.

•**Chinese herbs.** The formula contains a blend of six Chinese herbs—the most well-known is ginger, which often is used to treat upper-respiratory and sinus infections.

•**Echinacea.** Studies are mixed about this herb's benefit for the common cold. It appears, however, that certain standardized versions, such as the type used in Airborne, are quite effective.

•**Vitamin A.** Each Airborne tablet contains 5,000 international units (IU) of vitamin A, which is a therapeutic dose for supporting immune function. I have found the temporary use of vitamin A at doses above 10,000 IU per day to be effective for upper-respiratory tract infections. Vitamin A is used in the production of antibodies by the immune system. Pregnant women should not use vitamin A (at a dose above 5,000 IU daily) due to the risk of birth defects—therefore, they should avoid taking Airborne.

•**Minerals.** Small amounts of minerals also are found in Airborne, but they likely have only mild benefits. The most useful one is zinc, which enhances immune function. Airborne contains 8 mg of zinc per tablet, which is a sufficient dosage.

Overall, I think Airborne is worth using for the treatment of colds and as an added precaution, particularly when flying. It is reasonably priced at $5 for 10 tablets. Airborne's blend of herbs and nutrients likely enhances immune function. The product can be purchased at health-food and vitamin stores. A variety of flavors are available, as well as a children's formulation.

At the first sign of a cold, start taking an Airborne tablet every three waking hours for six days.

Ginseng Improves Cognitive Performance

I just read a very interesting study about mental performance. It involved 30 healthy young adults who first completed a 10-minute baseline test involving cognitive function and visual testing. Then they were given either 200 mg or 400 mg of standardized Panax (Asian or Chinese) ginseng or a placebo. One hour after the treatment, the participants took six more similar reasoning and visual tests in immediate succession.

The researchers found that Panax ginseng improved cognitive performance and mental alertness during sustained mental activity. The most notable effects were associated with the 200-mg dose. This benefit may be related to the significant reductions in blood glucose levels that were found in those taking ginseng. Blood glucose is the key fuel for brain-cell energy production—a reduction in blood glucose indicates that glucose is getting into the cells, in particular the brain cells, and is being used as fuel.

Ginseng can be taken once each morning. I recommend it for those who suffer from fatigue, poor concentration or high levels of stress as well as people with diabetes.

People with high blood pressure or those who take blood-thinning medications, such as *warfarin* (coumadin), and pregnant and nursing

113

women should not take ginseng. It is best not to take this stimulating herb in the evening because it may aggravate insomnia.

Should You Get a Flu Shot?

Every flu season, the government and much of the medical community promote flu vaccinations for millions of Americans. Should you get the vaccine? Here's what you need to know to make your decision.

There are two types of vaccines…

The "flu shot" contains inactive (killed) virus. The Centers for Disease Control and Prevention (CDC) says that it can be given to anyone over six months of age, including healthy people, pregnant and nursing women and those with chronic medical conditions.

The other form is a nasal-spray vaccine called FluMist. It contains attenuated (weakened) live viruses and should be used only by healthy people. Because FluMist involves live viruses, it should not be used by those who come in contact with people who have severely suppressed immune systems (such as transplant recipients or AIDS patients).

In addition, according to the CDC, the nasal-spray vaccine should not be used by…

- **Children younger than five years of age.**
- **People age 50 and older.**
- **People with a medical condition that places them at high risk for complications** from influenza, including those with chronic heart or lung disease, such as asthma or reactive airway disease…those with medical conditions such as diabetes or kidney failure…and those with illnesses that weaken the immune system—or anyone who takes medications that can weaken the immune system.
- **Children or adolescents taking aspirin.**
- **People with a history of Guillain-Barré syndrome,** a rare disorder that affects the nervous system.
- **Pregnant or nursing women.**

- **People with a history of allergy** to any of the components of the vaccine or to eggs.

Aside from the fact that some people get flu symptoms after getting the injected or nasal-spray vaccine, one of my biggest problems with the flu shot is that it contains *thimerosal,* a preservative that contains mercury.

Mercury is a known immune-system suppressant and is toxic to the nervous system. In my opinion, it can be particularly harmful to pregnant women because it exposes the fetus to mercury. Infants are not able to detoxify mercury effectively, and it can cause nerve and brain damage in children.

Some scientific evidence shows that thimerosal in vaccines leads to health problems, so in 1999, the US Public Health Service and the American Academy of Pediatrics—along with vaccine manufacturers—agreed that thimerosal should be reduced or eliminated in vaccines as a precaution. It has since been removed from childhood vaccines, yet manufacturers still are using thimerosal in the adult flu vaccine.

However, a preservative-free vaccine in a single-dose syringe is available. It contains only trace amounts of thimerosal as a residual from early manufacturing steps. Thimerosal is used as a preservative in an amount less than 1 mcg mercury/0.5 mL dose, versus the regular injectable version that contains 25 mcg mercury/0.5 mL dose. Ask your doctor about it if you are getting a shot.

For those who have a choice between types of flu vaccine, I recommend FluMist, which contains no mercury and often is available at pharmacies without a prescription.

The flu can be life-threatening for some people. For that reason, if you have risk factors for developing complications from the flu (see below) and aren't eligible to use FluMist, I recommend that you consider getting a preservative-free flu shot in October or November. *If a preservative-free vaccine is not available to you, you should still get a flu shot if you fall into any of the following groups…*

- **Anyone age 65 and older.**
- **Residents of nursing homes** or other long-term-care facilities that house people of any age who have chronic medical conditions.

114

•**Anyone who suffers from chronic disorders of the pulmonary or cardiovascular system.**

•**Anyone who has required regular medical follow-up or hospitalization during the preceding year** because of chronic metabolic diseases (including diabetes), renal dysfunction, blood cell disorders or immunosuppression (including that caused by medications or by human immunodeficiency virus, also known as HIV).

•**Children and adolescents ages six months to 18 years who are receiving long-term aspirin therapy** and, therefore, might be at risk for experiencing Reye's syndrome after influenza infection.

•**Children ages six months to 23 months.**

•**Women who will be pregnant during the influenza season.**

For my healthy patients, I recommend focusing on the powerful, natural cold-and-flu–fighting strategies discussed earlier in this issue, rather than vaccination.

THE POSSIBILITY OF A FLU PANDEMIC

Experts now are concerned about a global flu epidemic (pandemic) that could kill millions around the world—and it is quite possible. Consider the three influenza pandemics of the 20th century...

The Spanish flu of 1918 affected 20% to 40% of the world's population and killed more than 50 million people—675,00 people died in the US alone. The 1957 Asian flu pandemic resulted in approximately 70,000 deaths, and many still remember the 1968 Hong Kong flu that took the lives of more than 34,000 Americans.

In August 2004, Tommy G. Thompson, then Secretary of the US Department of Health and Human Services, unveiled the department's Pandemic Influenza Response and Preparedness Plan, which outlines a coordinated national strategy to prepare for and respond to an influenza pandemic. "This plan will serve as our road map on how we, as a nation and as a member of the global health community, respond to the next pandemic influenza outbreak, whenever that may be," he said at the time.

The US recently has been stockpiling flu vaccines, yet these are not likely to be of much help.

Influenza (and other viruses) constantly change their structure just enough so that the immune system doesn't recognize them. The mutation of viruses makes it difficult for manufacturers to predict which flu strain (out of the many hundreds) will make its way to the US.

Flu vaccines are manufactured several months before flu season actually begins, so they may not be accurate at all for the incoming influenza strain. With a pandemic influenza virus, there is a sudden change in the structure of the virus, that makes the manufacture of a vaccine nearly impossible.

According to a Department of Health and Human Services press release, "Pandemic virus will likely be unaffected by currently available flu vaccines that are modified each year to match the strains of the virus that are known to be in circulation among humans around the world."

Normally, changes occur gradually in the influenza viruses that appear. A pandemic influenza virus is particularly dangerous due to the major, sudden shift that is seen in the virus's structure. This increases the pandemic influenza virus's ability to cause illness in a large proportion of the population.

What is your best defense? A supercharged immune system that's ready to do battle with these viral intruders.

Beat Bad Breath

About half of Americans have bad breath (halitosis). Fortunately, a simple natural approach often is all it takes to eradicate the problem.

Several conditions may contribute to bad breath, including gum disease, degrading silver fillings, chronic dental and/or throat infections and ulcers and other digestive problems. It is important to work with your dentist to determine the cause because bad breath may indicate a bigger problem. *If your dentist can't find a problem, try these suggestions...*

Take one teaspoon of liquid *chlorophyll* (the green pigment in plants) straight or diluted in a glass of water after meals. Chlorophyll (available at most health-food stores) freshens breath immediately and supports detoxification of the digestive tract.

Many people who have bad breath have an overgrowth of bacteria in the mouth, which is typically caused by certain foods, sugar, lack of good bacteria and/or infection. For these cases, I recommend rinsing with *xylitol,* a natural sugar alcohol found in many fruits, berries, vegetables and mushrooms. Xylitol prevents bacteria from adhering to teeth and gums. I have seen good results with a product called Spry Coolmint Oral Rinse, which should be used twice daily. A 16-ounce bottle sells for $5. It is available at many health-food stores and some dentists' offices.

Arm Support Prevents Computer Injuries

People who use computers for long hours are at risk for strains and pains in the muscles and joints of the upper body. Researchers from the University of California, San Francisco, evaluated the effects of using a wide U-shaped board attached to the desk to support both forearms from elbow to wrist. Among the 182 participants, those using the arm board experienced 50% fewer neck and shoulder problems, and significantly less pain, than those who did not use the arm support.

My view: A surface that supports both forearms (rather than one or both wrists) allows muscles to relax while maintaining alignment of the neck, shoulders and arms. Arm supports are available from R&D Ergonomics (from $93.95, 800-813-7274, *www.morencyrest.com*).

A Daily Dose of Regularity

Taking daily magnesium supplements in excess of 800 mg can improve bowel regularity in the short term, but they may lead to poor nutrient absorption and nutritional deficiencies. This also can occur with long-term use of commercial laxatives.

Instead, promote regularity by eating more high-fiber foods, including vegetables, fruits, nuts, seeds and whole grains...drinking 64 ounces of water daily...and exercising regularly. If constipation persists, check a health-food store for psyllium seed husk powder—a source of insoluble fiber that softens stools.

Also helpful: A traditional Indian formula called *triphala* (composed of three fruits that stimulate intestinal contractions), such as Triphala Gold by Planetary Herbals (800-606-6226, *www.plane taryherbals.com*). If constipation continues for more than eight weeks, or if you develop abdominal pain or pencil-thin stools, see your doctor to get tested for bowel disease, underactive thyroid and other possible causes.

Drugs Can Be Custom-Made for You

Most pharmacies sell ready-made drugs. Compounding pharmacies, however, offer a distinct advantage—they provide prescription medications that are tailor-made for the individual.

Advantages: Dosage can be adjusted for body weight...patients with a history of adverse drug reactions can start with small doses and gradually build up, or they can obtain medications made without allergy-provoking preservatives and dyes...for convenience, several drugs may be combined into one formulation...and compounded drugs are less likely to degrade, because they are not made months in advance. Also, there may be more options for how compounded drugs are administered—such as capsules, skin patches or creams, rectal or vaginal suppositories, sublingual (under the tongue) tablets or troches (lozenges absorbed through mucous membranes in the cheeks), and therapies delivered by inhalation, injection (into a muscle) or intravenously (into a vein). In price, compounded drugs generally are competitive with ready-made drugs and usually are covered by insurance. For a referral, contact the International Academy of Compounding Pharmacists (800-927-4227, *www.iacprx.org*).

SPECIAL REPORT #6:

Hidden Health Dangers: What You Don't Know Can Hurt You

Hidden Health Dangers: What You Don't Know Can Hurt You

Healing Outside the Box Of Mainstream Medicine

Almost invariably, new patients tell me, "Conventional medicine is not helping me. I'm here to try something different." Americans are waking up to the fact that most diseases can be helped or healed through natural medicine. Yet success requires that patients and their doctors "think outside the box" of mainstream medicine.

Healing sometimes takes more than an open mind, however. I'm often impressed by my patients who demonstrate dedication to a new lifestyle...perseverance despite setbacks...and courage to combat a discouraging prognosis. Here are the stories of four patients from whom I've learned invaluable lessons. I hope you find them inspiring, too.

LISTEN TO YOUR BODY

"I've lost track of how many different doctors I've seen in the past three years," said Nancy, 39, a real estate agent and mother of four. "They never agree on what's wrong, other than to imply that my problems are in my head. But I believe in listening to my body—and it's telling me that something isn't right."

Nancy had a daunting list of two dozen symptoms, including relentless fatigue, widespread muscle pain, dry skin, hair loss, weight gain, hypoglycemia (low blood sugar), recurring respiratory infections, dizzy spells, panic attacks and heart palpitations. Her various medical doctors had run numerous blood tests and other laboratory analyses over the years, but the results had always been "normal." Several times Nancy was offered antidepressants, which she refused. "I'm not sick because I'm depressed—I'm depressed because I'm sick," she told me.

Instead of trying to treat Nancy's symptoms one by one, I looked for a connection among

---

Mark A. Stengler, ND, naturopathic physician in private practice, La Jolla, California...adjunct associate clinical professor at the National College of Natural Medicine, Portland, Oregon...author of many books, including *The Natural Physician's Healing Therapies* and coauthor of *Prescription for Natural Cures* (both from Bottom Line Books)...and author of the *Bottom Line/Natural Healing* newsletter.

her seemingly disparate problems—and recognized that many of them suggested low thyroid function. I ordered a blood test for *free T3*, the most specific marker of thyroid function available. (T3 is one of the thyroid hormones, and the "free" level is the amount not bound to protein and therefore available for use by the body's cells.) This test is not routinely ordered by most doctors, though I think it should be used more often.

The test confirmed that Nancy's free T3 level was low. I prescribed Armour Thyroid, a brand of natural thyroid hormone in tablet form that contains T3 and a blend of other thyroid hormones found in the human body. Most thyroid prescriptions do not contain T3, but instead contain only T4, a less potent and less effective thyroid hormone.

The results were fantastic. Within one week, Nancy's fatigue had eased and her mood had improved. Over the next three months, her energy level returned to normal...muscle pain disappeared...respiratory infections cleared up... weight and blood sugar stabilized...skin and hair condition improved...and mood lifted. Nancy said, "I can hardly believe how well I feel from just one simple type of treatment."

Self-help strategy: Before seeing a dozen different specialists for a dozen different symptoms, consult a holistic doctor. He/she will evaluate you as a whole person, rather than as a collection of problematic body parts—and may identify a single root cause behind all your symptoms. A good holistic doctor also will acknowledge that you know your own body best and will take all your concerns seriously.

HELP CELLS TO HELP THEMSELVES

A dedicated farmer and proud new grandparent, David was devastated when his oncologist reported that his prostate cancer had spread to his breastbone and that chemotherapy could not help. In an attempt to keep the cancer from spreading further, David underwent radiation treatments. He also received injections of drugs to reduce his body's production of testosterone and estrogen, since these hormones are associated with prostate cancer. Despite these measures, his prognosis was bleak. "Get your affairs in order," his doctor advised. "You've got about 12 months." David was 55 years old.

Though he had never given credence to alternative medicine, David decided that he had nothing to lose. At his son-in-law's urging, he came to see me.

I emphasized the need for David to help his cells detoxify—to release toxins that could be causing the cancer and to minimize the harmful side effects of the radiation treatments. I also recommended that we stimulate his immune system so that it could more effectively combat the disease.

First line of defense: A detoxifying diet, a topic I covered in the April 2006 issue of *Natural Healing.**

Although he had been a lifelong beef lover, frequent beer drinker and occasional cake baker, David immediately gave up red meat, alcohol and sugary foods, and greatly increased his intake of nutritious vegetables and fish. He also began taking daily supplements of cancer-fighting vitamin C and selenium...the herbal detoxifiers dandelion root, burdock root and milk thistle... and various natural immune boosters, including echinacea and Oregon grape root.

The nutrients did their job better than David had dared to hope. He is now cancer-free—10 years after his doctor had predicted his imminent demise. David remains conscientious about his detoxifying diet-and-supplement regimen. "It's the reason I'm here today," he says, "watching my grandson grow up."

Self-help strategy: By detoxifying the body, it's often possible to fight serious diseases at the most basic cellular level. By being open-minded about alternative therapies, you expand your treatment options and optimize healing.

SAY NO TO DRUGS...AND YES TO NUTRITION

Victor, 12, was in trouble at school. For years, the the boy's behavior had caused problems in the classroom, and recently his restlessness and outbursts had worsened. His grades, never good, had dropped perilously close to failing. After Victor's pediatrician diagnosed attention deficit-hyperactivity disorder (ADHD), the school psychologist and principal pressured the boy's parents, warning, "If Victor does not go

*For a free copy of the article, go to *www.BottomLine Secrets.com/SpringCleaning*, or send a self-addressed, stamped envelope to "Spring Cleaning," Boardroom Inc., Box 412, Stamford, Connecticut 06904-0412.

on ADHD medication, he will be asked to leave the school."

But Victor's mother stood firm—"Those drugs can have serious side effects. We need to explore all other options first." That's when the family contacted me.

I shared the family's concerns about ADHD drugs, such as *methylphenidate* (Ritalin) and *amphetamine/dextroamphetamine* (Adderall XR), which can cause nausea, loss of appetite and stunted growth...headaches, dizziness and tics...insomnia and fatigue...irritability and mood swings...and heart palpitations, blood pressure changes and an increased risk of heart attack. We agreed to try nutritional therapies first and to use drugs only as a last resort.

Fortunately, we had summer vacation to address Victor's problems. The boy's diet was already good—but nonetheless, I suspected a deficiency of *essential fatty acids* (EFAs), which are vital structural components of cell membranes that affect the health of the brain, nervous system and cardiovascular system.

The clue: Victor's skin was extremely dry. EFA deficiency is a common cause of dry skin, and studies show that EFA supplementation improves mood and focus in some children with ADHD.

To boost Victor's intake of EFAs, I started him on daily supplements of fish oil (Nordic Naturals Pro DHA, 800-662-2544, *www.nordicnaturals. com*) and evening primrose oil. In addition, I prescribed the homeopathic remedy *Lycopodium clavatum*, made from club moss, to improve mood and concentration. I also had Victor take daily supplements of *phosphatidylserine*—a nutrient essential for the normal functioning of brain cell membranes and naturally found in soy, rice, fish and leafy green vegetables.

Victor was tested by a child psychologist before starting his treatment with me and again after 10 weeks. To the psychologist's amazement, Victor improved so markedly that he was no longer considered to have ADHD. During the ensuing school year, his teachers reported that Victor's behavior was exemplary. When I asked the boy during a follow-up visit, "How are your grades?" he grinned from ear to ear as he answered, "I made the honor roll!"

Self-help strategy: Many behavioral problems result from biochemical imbalances. Before resorting to drugs, investigate potential side effects—and explore natural alternatives that can safely restore the body's proper balance.

PERSEVERANCE PAYS OFF

Turning 40, Joanne laughed at the idea of a midlife crisis. She was happily married and had a busy, successful medical practice as a doctor of chiropractic. Life was good, and the future looked bright.

But then Joanne began to experience recurring pain in her bladder and the surrounding pelvic area, plus a frequent and urgent need to urinate. Her doctor diagnosed interstitial cystitis (IC), a condition that affects more than 700,000 people in the US (primarily women), yet is still not well understood. Joanne tried every treatment her doctors could suggest—including the prescription drug *pentosan polysulfate* (Elmiron), which is intended to repair the bladder lining, and a surgical procedure called bladder distension, which stretches the bladder by filling it with gas or water to increase its capacity—but nothing brought relief.

After five years, Joanne was in such severe and incessant pain that she could no longer see patients, take care of her two-year-old or find any pleasure in sex. Compounding her problems, she also experienced an early menopause, with symptoms that included dozens of hot flashes a day, frequent insomnia and severe fatigue, heart palpitations, anxiety, mood swings and trouble concentrating.

As I took her medical history, I noticed that her IC symptoms had eased during her pregnancy. This suggested that her IC was connected to her hormone balance and that menopause was aggravating the condition. Blood and saliva tests confirmed that she had a deficiency of estrogen, progesterone and thyroid hormones.

Finding the root of Joanne's problem was easier than treating it. For seven months, we used a trial-and-error approach, looking for a precise mix of hormone replacement therapies to alleviate her IC and menopausal symptoms. Finally, we hit upon the solution—a mix of an *estriol* (estrogen) vaginal cream...an estrogen/progesterone combination transdermal (skin) cream...and oral thyroid hormone tablets. Two months later,

Joanne's pelvic pain and urinary urgency were gone, her menopausal symptoms had abated, and her sex life was back on track. "I'm enjoying being a mom," she reported, "and I may reopen my chiropractic practice. I've got my life back!"

Self-help strategy: Joanne deserves credit for her patience as we worked to figure out the best treatment for her individual needs. Too many people give up if they don't find a quick fix. For health problems—as with most of life's challenges—perseverance is the key to finding a solution.

When You Need Support

Facing a medical problem? Reach out for help. These organizations can provide physician referrals...information on conditions, treatments and research...and/or emotional support.

COMPLEMENTARY AND ALTERNATIVE MEDICINE

•**American Association of Naturopathic Physicians,** 866-538-2267, *www.naturopathic. org.*

•**American Association of Acupuncture and Oriental Medicine,** 866-455-7999, *www. aaaomonline.org.*

•**American College for Advancement in Medicine,** 800-532-3688, *www.acamnet.org.*

•**National Center for Homeopathy,** 703-548-7790, *www.nationalcenterforhomeopathy.org.*

MAINSTREAM MEDICINE

•**American Autoimmune Related Diseases Association,** 202-466-8511, *www.aarda.org.*

•**American Cancer Society,** 800-227-2345, *www.cancer.org.*

•**American Diabetes Association,** 800-342-2383, *www.diabetes.org.*

•**American Heart Association,** 800-242-8721, *www.americanheart.org.*

•**American Lung Association,** 800-586-4872, *www.lungusa.org.*

•**National Alliance on Mental Illness,** 800-950-6264, *www.nami.org.*

Is Fish Really That Good for You?

If you're a fish eater, as I am, you may be questioning whether or not you should still eat it. You have no doubt heard that fish can be loaded with contaminants, particularly mercury, and you may be wondering if the risks of eating fish outweigh the health benefits.

Fish do indeed provide a range of health benefits. They are high in protein but relatively low in calories, saturated fat and cholesterol. They also are an excellent source of omega-3 fatty acids. These good fats are important for cardiovascular health. They improve blood flow by regulating blood vessel constriction, and they have blood-thinning properties that help prevent strokes.

In addition, omega-3s reduce inflammatory responses—important for preventing not only heart disease but also Alzheimer's disease, various cancers, osteoarthritis and rheumatoid arthritis.

MERCURY DANGER

Unfortunately, some fish have become so loaded with contaminants that they pose health risks, especially when consumed too frequently. One of these contaminants is mercury, which is toxic to the brain as well as the nervous and immune systems.

Mercury occurs naturally in trace amounts in the environment, but because of industrial pollution, high concentrations of mercury have accumulated in lakes, rivers and oceans. In the water, mercury is converted by bacteria into an organic form known as methylmercury. Small fish eat aquatic organisms that have consumed *methylmercury*. Larger fish eat the smaller fish, and methylmercury makes its way up the food chain. Fish do not eliminate methylmercury efficiently, and it builds up in their bodies.

Larger fish, such as shark, swordfish, tilefish and king mackerel, contain the highest amounts of methylmercury. The US Food and Drug Administration (FDA) advises pregnant women, women who might become pregnant, nursing mothers and children to avoid these fish. I support this recommendation for everyone because I believe that mercury toxicity is more of a problem than is recognized by the FDA.

IS TUNA SAFE?

My patients commonly ask me if canned tuna is safe to eat. The two most popular types are chunk white and light tuna. Canned chunk white tuna is made from albacore, a large species of tuna that contains moderate levels of mercury. Canned light tuna is usually made of skipjack, a smaller species that has about 40% less mercury than albacore. I do not recommend the consumption of white tuna at all. Light tuna should be limited to six ounces every two weeks, but it should not be consumed by children or pregnant women.

Certain brands of tuna have lower amounts of mercury. One example is Oregon's Choice Gourmet (877-289-8862, *www.oregonschoice.com*).

There is no difference in mercury levels between tuna packed in water and tuna in oil, but water-packed tuna contains more omega-3s because oil leaches out some of these healthful fatty acids.

Yellowfin, bigeye and bluefin tuna are commonly used for sushi and sashimi. They have high mercury levels and should be avoided (for an exception, see "Best Choices" below).

BEST CHOICES

It may sound like there are no safe fish, but there are some you can eat without much concern. Wild salmon (which I think is more healthful than the farmed variety), anchovies, Atlantic herring, sardines and tilapia are good choices. The Web site *www.oceansalive.org*—maintained by the Environmental Defense Network, a nonprofit organization—provides an excellent rating system of the best and worst seafood choices for health.

There are safe options for tuna as well. This past March, I lectured at the Natural Products Expo West convention, which features health industry supplements and foods. During my free time, I wandered through the more than 3,000 exhibits. One that caught both my wife Angela's and my attention was a company from Hawaii named Kona Blue.

Kona Blue has come up with one way to control contamination of its tuna. The company raises a type of sushi-grade Hawaiian yellowtail known as Kona Kampachi (*Seriola rivoliana*). I like yellowtail sushi but rarely eat it because it tends to be high in mercury. Not this yellowtail.

Kona Kampachi has no detectable mercury or PCBs, and the company does not use antibiotics. The tuna are raised in their natural habitat in large, submerged cages in the clean open ocean a half mile off the coast of the big island of Hawaii.

Kona Blue's Hawaiian yellowtail is especially rich in omega-3 fatty acids, with approximately 2.95 g of omega-3s per 100 g of fish, including any water present in the fish's tissues. By comparison, Atlantic mackerel has 2.45 g, Atlantic salmon has 1.73 g, albacore tuna 1.5 g and halibut 0.42 g.

Hawaii has the oldest tradition of aquaculture in the US. It was first practiced by the Polynesians who settled on the islands more than 1,000 years ago. Ancient Hawaiians raised fish and crab in coastal ponds created by stone walls and connected to the ocean.

According to the Hawaii Department of Agriculture, there are more than 100 aquafarms in Hawaii, which raise such shellfish as marine shrimp, freshwater prawns, abalone…finfish, such as Pacific threadfin or moi, tilapia, catfish, carp, flounder, sturgeon, amberjack, snapper and grouper…and various types of algae, including seaweed, and microalgae, such as spirulina (a popular nutritional supplement). This type of approach is exactly what is needed when almost half the world's fisheries are depleted from overfishing, and many species are on the brink of extinction.

The Kona Kampachi yellowtail has a smooth texture and a rich taste. Angela and I both enjoyed sampling it. It is available at retail markets, including Whole Foods, and is served in sushi restaurants across the country.

To find out where it's available in your area or to order the fish directly, go to the Web site *www.kona-blue.com* or call 877-875-1188. The mail-order retail price per pound is $17 for fillets and $8.75 for whole fish. It is shipped via Fedex, and it is recommended that someone be available to accept delivery and refrigerate the fish immediately.

Can Bread Make You Sick? The Answer Is Yes!

Millions of people endure chronic symptoms including abdominal pain and bouts of fatigue—but they don't have to.

For you (or someone you love), the solution to these and many other troubles might be shockingly simple—*if* you and your doctor are willing to do a little unusual sleuthing.

When Bonita, age 60, came to see me, she complained of daily abdominal pain and flatulence. She told me that she had suffered frequent waves of fatigue since she was a child. Numerous visits to doctors and specialists over the years turned up a variety of problems. Bonita had been diagnosed with chronic anemia (low red blood cell count) and hypoglycemia (low blood sugar). Those conditions could help account for her fatigue.

There were other issues as well. Osteoporosis had set in—a bone density scan showed loss of bone mass. Bonita also had lost too much weight. Examinations revealed that she also had fatty liver (fat buildup in the liver cells) and inflammation of the pancreas. Typically, when I see such signs in the liver and pancreas, I suspect excessive alcohol consumption—but Bonita didn't touch a drop!

These signs pointed to celiac disease (CD), also sometimes called by its older name, sprue. If you don't know much about this condition, you're not alone. It took medical researchers many years to unravel its root cause—and even today, lots of people have it and don't know it.

When I ran some additional blood tests on Bonita, my suspicions proved correct. I immediately put her on a diet free of gluten (a protein complex found in wheat, barley and rye), meaning she could have absolutely no bread, crackers, cake, cereal or other foods containing these common grains. Within weeks, there was a noticeable improvement in Bonita's energy. Her abdominal pain diminished. Blood tests showed that her anemia was improving, as were liver and pancreatic function. She felt much better, gained some weight and looked vibrant!

THE CURSE OF THE GRAIN

Celiac disease (CD), the cause of Bonita's life-long discomfort, is an autoimmune condition. This means that the immune system—designed to prevent infection and fight off disease—turns traitor and harms the body.

With CD, the body recognizes gluten as a harmful foreign substance. When someone with CD consumes gluten, a big problem develops in the small intestine—specifically with the multitude of soft, tiny, fingerlike projections called *villi* that line the intestinal walls. Villi are responsible for absorbing nutrients.

In people who have CD, the villi are damaged and can't do their job properly. They're caught in a cross fire between the immune system and the gluten that's traveling through the small intestine. For some reason, in certain people—this is the part we don't fully understand—the immune system attacks the gluten, and the fragile villi get mauled in the autoimmune battle.

When a CD sufferer stops eating foods that contain gluten, the turnaround can be remarkable—and often within a matter of weeks. For people who have suffered with this condition for years without knowing the cause, eliminating gluten can seem like the beginning of a new life.

Many doctors don't pay much attention to CD's all-too-common signs. That's a big mistake because recent studies have shown that it is much more prevalent than previously suspected. At a conference held by the National Institutes of Health in 2004, researchers reported that CD affects as many as 3 million Americans, or about one out of every 100 people.

MALABSORPTION MAYHEM

CD leaves plenty of clues. When inflamed villi can no longer absorb nutrients as they should, you end up with a condition called *malabsorption*, which results in nutritional deficiencies.

Other possible damage can occur as well, including a condition called *increased intestinal permeability*. This type of intestinal-wall damage can be compared to holes punched in a screen door—larger-than-normal molecules can escape through holes in the small intestine and enter the bloodstream. Among those larger molecules are portions of protein compounds (gluten fractions) that aren't supposed to penetrate the intestinal wall.

Result: The body, sensing the presence of these fractions, begins to intensify the autoimmune reaction.

If an infant or a child has CD, malabsorption takes a cruel toll. Some infants display signs of "failure to thrive" (slowed growth in a number of the body's systems). Older children may have physical and behavioral development problems.

The longer CD goes undetected and a person continues to eat gluten, the more likely he/she is to develop other autoimmune diseases—insulin-dependent type 1 diabetes, thyroiditis (inflammation of the thyroid) and hepatitis (inflammation of the liver). People with untreated CD also have an elevated risk of certain types of cancer, especially intestinal lymphoma. While CD exists in sufferers from birth through adulthood, the symptoms may start to show up at any time.

THE TESTS—WHAT'S INVOLVED?

CD can affect anyone, but it is more prevalent in people of European (especially Northern European) descent. Studies also show that it affects Hispanic, black and Asian populations.

Because neglecting CD can be life-threatening, I recommend that screening begin in early childhood. If you have any of the symptoms (see box) or suffer from lupus, type 1 diabetes, rheumatoid arthritis or thyroid disease, then it is even more critical to be screened for CD. Genetics is a factor, so if a parent, sibling or child of yours tests positive for CD, I recommend that you also get screened.

CD is detected by a group of blood tests referred to as a celiac panel. These tests, which generally are covered by health insurance, measure your immune system's response to gluten in the foods you eat. If blood tests point to a diagnosis of CD, your doctor may recommend that you see a gastroenterologist for a biopsy of the small intestine.

The biopsy involves the use of an endoscope (a long, thin tube with a tiny periscope and cutting tool at the end), which is inserted through the mouth and manipulated through the small intestine. If the extracted villi are severely damaged, it confirms CD.

Caution: Don't stop consuming gluten before a celiac blood test or biopsy. This could throw off your test results. (Fortunately, the blood tests now used to diagnose CD are so accurate that a biopsy usually isn't necessary.)

GLUTEN SENSITIVITY

If you have a number of symptoms that suggest CD but your test results are negative, there's a chance that you have a less severe form of the condition, called *gluten sensitivity*. In my own practice, I have found that gluten sensitivity is much more common than CD.

Some patients complain of bloating, headache, rashes or other symptoms that might be related to CD or to allergies, but traditional skin-scratch or blood antibody tests don't point to a single diagnosis. To find out whether gluten is a factor, I recommend reducing (or better, eliminating) intake of wheat and other gluten-containing grains. If symptoms improve, it's a strong indication of gluten sensitivity.

Some people with gluten sensitivity can eat grains as long as they "rotate" among different kinds—that is, consuming different grains instead of the same ones all the time—to reduce symptoms and provide a wider variety of nutrients. This plan is not appropriate for people who have CD—they must completely eliminate gluten from their diets, permanently, period.

WHAT THE FUTURE HOLDS

Continuing research shows that we still have much to learn about CD, but there is good reason to be hopeful that prevention might one day be possible. In identical twins who live in the same household, for example, sometimes only one has CD—raising the question of what role environment plays.

A study published in *American Journal of Clinical Nutrition* showed that the more gluten-containing foods introduced to an infant, the greater the risk of developing CD in childhood. However, breast-feeding during this time cuts the risk of developing CD in childhood. We don't yet know whether these findings hold true throughout life.

And, based on Dutch research, there may be a connection between the overgrowth of *Candida albicans*, a yeast normally found in the digestive tract, and the onset of CD, perhaps because of chemical similarities between *Candida* and gluten. The idea that infections of the gut and autoimmune conditions are linked continues to gain acceptance—and I will keep you up to date.

Wheat-Free, Worry-Free: The Art of Happy, Healthy, Gluten-Free Living, by Danna Korn (Hay House).

Going Against the Grain: How Reducing and Avoiding Grains Can Revitalize Your Health, by Melissa Diane Smith (McGraw Hill).

SIGNS OF CELIAC DISEASE (CD)

CD is associated with a wide range of symptoms, including…

- **Diarrhea**
- **Feeling or looking bloated**
- **Unexplained fatigue**
- **Unexplained abdominal pain**
- **Gassiness**
- **Skin redness, rash, itchy skin**
- **Loss of tooth enamel**
- **Unexpected hair loss**
- **Low body weight**
- **Infertility or irregular menses**
- **Premature osteoporosis**

If you have any of these symptoms, ask your doctor about CD—the sooner, the better.

How to Go Gluten-Free

As restricted diets go, gluten-free is not bad. You can eat meat, seafood, fruits and vegetables. There are no restrictions against nuts, peas, beans, soybeans and items made from them, such as tofu made from soybeans. You also are allowed to eat rice, corn and a variety of other grains, including amaranth, buckwheat (kasha), millet, quinoa and sorghum, and anything made from them, including rice pasta. In recent years, researchers have stated that oats also can be eaten. Dairy products, wine and sweets are safe, too. All of the above assumes that these foods haven't been processed or cooked with any gluten-containing ingredients.

Here's the slightly tricky part. In avoiding wheat and the other grains listed below, it's easy to forgo obvious gluten-containing foods, such as bread (and most things that are breaded), cookies, pancakes, etc. But you must watch out for the many food products that aren't grains per se but that contain gluten because they are made with grain derivatives, such as wheat starch or malt (from barley). Less obvious gluten-containing ingredients are commonly used in condiments…sauces (including soy sauce)…salad dressings…meat products such as sausage and cold cuts… processed seafood products…processed cheese products…etc. Even some dietary supplements and medications contain gluten. The basic rule with CD is, when in doubt, don't eat it. Call the manufacturer to find out for next time.

Now more good news. The food industry is waking up to CD, and you will find a growing number of gluten-free cooking ingredients. Many chain supermarkets now have a gluten-free section. Even restaurants are starting to offer gluten-free choices, and several national chains—including Legal Sea Foods, Outback Steakhouse and PF Chang's China Bistro—have developed gluten-free menus.

For more on gluten-free eating, go to the Celiac Disease Foundation's site, *www.celiac.org,* and the Celiac Sprue Association's site, *www. csaceliacs.org.*

FOODS TO AVOID

- **Wheat,** including wheat flour, wheat germ, wheat bran, cracked wheat, einkorn wheat, emmer wheat
  - **Couscous**
  - **Kamut**
  - **Spelt**
  - **Semolina**
  - **Rye**
  - **Triticale** (wheat-rye hybrid)
  - **Barley**

Nontoxic Cleaning

Do you suffer from unexplained headaches, breathing problems (asthma or burning of the airway), mood swings and/or skin rashes? These and other chronic problems may be related to the cleansers you use in your home. Common ingredients include ammonia and chlorine (both skin and lung irritants), *formaldehyde* (an irritant to the nervous system and a suspected carcinogen) and *trisodium nitrilotriacetate* (a suspected carcinogen).

You should be particularly concerned if there are infants or young children in the home—developing bodies are more susceptible to injury from toxic substances than those of adults. In my home, we use nontoxic, biodegradable cleansers, from laundry detergents to disinfectants. Much of household cleaning and laundry can be done using inexpensive, safe and natural ingredients—baking soda, lemon juice, vinegar, borax and vegetable soaps, such as coconut, Castile or beeswax soap.

Look for products that are biodegradable, nontoxic, recyclable and nonpetroleum-derived with a phosphate concentration of 0.5% or less by weight. This information should appear on the manufacturers' Web sites. Seventh Generation carries a complete line of nontoxic household products (to find a retailer, call 800-456-1191, *www.seventh generation.com*) as does Earth Friendly Products (800-335-3267, *www.ecos.com*). Both brands work very well.

Cooked Broccoli and Thyroid Function

I have advised readers and patients to avoid cooking broccoli, but this may not be the best way to go if you have thyroid problems.

Broccoli contains *goitrogens*, substances that can interfere with the function of the thyroid gland. Other foods that contain goitrogens include brussels sprouts, cabbage, cauliflower, kale, kohlrabi, mustard greens, rutabagas and turnips, as well as soy, millet, peaches, peanuts, radishes and spinach.

There is little data on the effect of these foods on human thyroid function. I advised readers to eat broccoli raw or lightly steamed and avoid boiling it so it doesn't lose its vitamin C and phytonutrient content. But I recommend that people with existing thyroid problems, especially low thyroid function (hypothyroidism), or

those with a family history of hypothyroidism, consume these foods raw only in moderation (a maximum of two to three servings a week will give you the full benefit of the food's vitamin C and phytonutrients). Cooking these foods appears to inactivate the goitrogens, allowing you to eat them more than two or three times a week if you choose to do so.

Cholesterol Mania— Stop Taking Drugs You Don't Need

Cholesterol-lowering "statin" drugs are big business. *Atorvastatin* (Lipitor), one of the most popular drugs in this class, is among the most commonly prescribed medications in the US. With approximately 12 million Americans using it, US sales of Lipitor totaled about $8 billion in 2005.

Why are so many people taking these drugs? It's long been known that elevated cholesterol levels are associated with an increased risk of heart disease, but now consumers are being given an additional incentive to use these drugs. The National Institutes of Health's National Cholesterol Education Program (NCEP) Adult Treatment Panel III recently released updated guidelines for cholesterol drug therapy. According to these guidelines, 37 million Americans—or one in five adults—are eligible for cholesterol-lowering medication. Previous guidelines recommended these drugs for 13 million Americans. I find the new guidelines very suspect. Read on, and you will understand why.

The updated recommendations are based on a review of five clinical trials using statins. One of the key changes in the new guidelines involved lowering the optimal range for LDL "bad" cholesterol in the blood in all adults to less than 100 milligrams per deciliter (mg/dL). People with cardiovascular disease or other risk factors, such as diabetes, smoking or hypertension, are told to aim for the same level—with an "optional target" of less than 70 mg/dL. It is rare for any of the patients I test—whether they are healthy or not—to have LDL levels below 100 mg/dL. I encourage my patients to strive for an LDL level of 100 mg/dL to 130 mg/dL with an HDL "good" cholesterol level of 50 mg/dL or higher.

The evidence for the recent NCEP guidelines was challenged in a letter from the Center for Science in the Public Interest (CSPI), a nonprofit consumer advocacy group that conducts research in health and nutrition.

The CSPI letter, which was signed by more than three dozen physicians, epidemiologists and other scientists, urged the NIH to convene an independent panel to conduct a second review of the studies. They wrote, "There is strong evidence to suggest that an objective, independent reevaluation of the scientific evidence from the five new studies of statin therapy would lead to different conclusions than those presented by the current NCEP. The studies cited do not demonstrate that statins benefit women of any age or men over 70 who do not already have heart disease."

The letter also cited concerns that were raised after one study showed that statin therapy significantly *increases* the risk of some types of cancer in the elderly. (Research has, indeed, shown that statins can increase risk of nonmelanoma skin cancer and breast cancer. Other research, however, has linked statin use to a decreased risk for some types of cancer, such as colon and prostate malignancies.)

There was another alarming discovery. Eight of the nine authors of the new LDL recommendations had financial ties to statin drug manufacturers, including Pfizer, Merck, Bristol-Myers Squibb and AstraZeneca. In response to the CSPI letter, the NIH declared that the scientific basis for the new guidelines was adequate and there was no conflict of interest for panel members.

No conflict? Is it pure coincidence that most of the authors of the guidelines had financial ties to statin manufacturers? Now millions of Americans are following these misguided recommendations for statin therapy instead of using natural treatments.

UNDERSTANDING THE DANGERS OF STATINS

Statins first became available in the US in the late 1980s, when they were marketed as a unique treatment for elevated cholesterol—they inhibit an enzyme called *3-hydroxymethylglutaryl-coenzyme A* (HMG-CoA) reductase, which is involved in the production of cholesterol in the liver. In addition to Lipitor, other statins include *rosuvastatin* (Crestor), *lovastatin* (Mevacor), *pravastatin* (Pravachol) and *simvastatin* (Zocor).

The most common side effects of statins are headache, nausea, vomiting, constipation, diarrhea, rash, weakness, muscle and joint pain and increased liver enzymes. The most serious, but rare, side effects are liver failure and rhabdomyolysis, a life-threatening condition that causes extensive damage to muscles.

In addition, statins deplete the body of coenzyme Q10 (CoQ10), a naturally occurring substance that your body needs to create energy in cells, particularly heart cells. In one study, the CoQ10 blood levels of Lipitor users were reduced by 50% after 30 days of statin use. To prevent a deficiency of CoQ10, I recommend that my patients who use statins take 100 mg to 200 mg daily of CoQ10.

CHOLESTEROL-LOWERING THE NATURAL WAY

The general medical community pays lip service to diet and lifestyle changes as a first line of therapy for abnormal cholesterol levels—but many patients are pressured to begin drug therapy right away, while diet and lifestyle changes are only an afterthought. Conventional doctors often tell patients that they have a genetic cholesterol problem and that cholesterol-lowering medication is their only option because diet and lifestyle changes would not be sufficient. Some people, such as those who have acute cardiovascular issues or extremely high total cholesterol levels (above 350 mg/dL) and/or significantly elevated LDL levels (above 200 mg/dL), are usually not able to control their cholesterol levels through diet and lifestyle changes alone. However, many people can bring their cholesterol and lipid levels into normal range by watching what they eat, exercising and reducing their stress levels. Nutritional supplements also are an option.

If your cholesterol is mildly or moderately elevated (total cholesterol 200 mg/dL to 239 mg/dL...and/or LDL above 130 mg/dL), get a baseline cholesterol test if your levels haven't been tested in the last six months. Then try the diet and lifestyle changes described in this article for eight to 12 weeks.

People who are unable to reduce their cholesterol levels through diet and exercise and/or who have family members with high cholesterol *are* likely to be genetically predisposed to the condition. Such people should *not* rely on lifestyle changes alone.

Better: They should combine the healthful practices described here with regular supplement use.

Important: There are times when I recommend statin therapy—immediately after a heart attack to reduce inflammation and when there is extreme elevation in total cholesterol (400 mg/dL or higher) and/or LDL cholesterol (210 mg/dL or higher), usually due to genetics.

DIET AND LIFESTYLE CHANGES

My top suggestions for improving cholesterol levels…

1. Reduce saturated fat in your diet to less than 7% of daily calories. Saturated fat is found mainly in beef, veal, pork and poultry (especially in dark meat and the skin of any meat). Saturated fat is plentiful in most dairy products, except nonfat yogurt, reduced-fat cheese and skimmed milk. Small amounts are found in coconut and palm oils, so consume these sparingly. To monitor your saturated fat intake, keep a daily record based on food label information.

Avoid products that contain trans fatty acids, which often are found in deep-fried foods, bakery products, packaged snack foods, margarines (except those with cholesterol-reducing plant stanols or plant sterols), crackers and vegetable shortening. If a product contains more than 0.5 grams of trans fat per serving, the label will list the trans fat content. Avoid foods that "hide" trans fats by using the term "partially hydrogenated" on their labels and claiming 0 grams (g) of trans fat. Common offenders include baked goods, crackers and packaged mixes. Cardiovascular disease is linked to trans fat intake because this unhealthful fat raises levels of LDL cholesterol and blood fats known as triglycerides, while lowering beneficial HDL cholesterol. Cook with organic olive or canola oil. Macadamia nut oil also is healthful.

2. Consume two weekly servings of foods rich in heart-healthy omega-3 fatty acids. Sources include some types of fish—anchovies, Atlantic herring, sardines, tilapia and wild or canned salmon. For a list of fish not contaminated with mercury or polychlorinated biphenyls (PCBs), check *www.oceansalive.org*, the Web site of The Environmental Defense Network, a Washington, DC-based, nonprofit group dedicated to solving environmental problems.

3. Eat five to seven daily servings of fruits and vegetables. Produce contains antioxidants that prevent oxidation (cell damage from negatively charged molecules known as free radicals) of cholesterol, as well as fiber that helps lower cholesterol.

4. Consume foods that contain soluble (dissolves in liquid) fiber, such as beans, barley, oats, peas, apples, oranges and pears. Soluble fiber reduces the absorption of cholesterol from the intestines into the bloodstream. For example, a daily bowl of oatmeal can reduce total cholesterol by as much as 23%. Oatmeal also has been shown to curb LDL cholesterol levels without lowering beneficial HDL cholesterol.

5. Eat nuts, such as walnuts and almonds, which are rich in healthful monounsaturated fatty acids. A study conducted in Barcelona, Spain, showed that a walnut-rich diet reduces total cholesterol by 4.4% and LDL cholesterol by 6.4%. Macadamia nuts, pistachios, almonds, hazelnuts and pecans also have been shown to reduce cholesterol levels. Eat a handful of walnuts or any of the nuts listed above daily.

6. Add ground flaxseed (up to one-quarter cup daily, taken in two doses) to protein shakes, cereal and/or salads. Flaxseed has been shown to reduce total and LDL cholesterol. Drink 10 ounces of water for every two tablespoons of flaxseed you consume, to prevent intestinal blockage.

7. Consume 20 g to 30 g of soy protein daily (in food or protein powder form). Some studies suggest that soy protein may lower cholesterol levels in some people with high cholesterol. Because soy protein has a potential estrogen-like effect, it should be avoided by women who have breast cancer or a family history of the disease.

8. Reduce daily intake of simple sugars, such as those in crackers, cookies and soda. Found in abundance in processed packaged foods and many baked goods, they have been shown to decrease HDL cholesterol. By cutting back, you also reduce risk of elevated insulin levels, which lead to increased production of cholesterol by the liver.

9. Exercise regularly. Thirty minutes of exercise, such as brisk walking, swimming, biking or tennis, three to five times a week is effective for lowering elevated cholesterol.

10. Lose weight and body fat. Weight loss by people who are overweight reduces cholesterol levels and prevents insulin resistance, a blood sugar problem that can lead to high cholesterol.

11. Don't smoke. Smokers have lower levels of HDL cholesterol and an increased risk of heart attacks.

12. Adopt stress-reduction techniques, such as deep breathing and biofeedback. Stress has been shown to elevate cholesterol in most individuals.

Ahhh…Safe, Quick Relief From Hemorrhoid Pain— You Don't Need Surgery!

"My hemorrhoids are driving me crazy," said Don, a 55-year-old man who recently visited me for a consultation. "The bleeding and itching have been really bad this year, so my doctor is recommending surgery. What do you think?"

I could tell that Don was desperate for relief, but I felt obligated to share my concerns about the procedure.

"Have you ever spoken with someone who has had hemorrhoid surgery?" I asked.

"Well, no," Don replied.

"Believe me, it's the last thing you want to consider," I said. "The pain can be excruciating for several days, or even weeks, afterward, and the hemorrhoids can return."

I presented Don with an alternative to surgery—he could change his diet, take nutritional supplements and get more exercise (physical activity improves circulation and promotes bowel regularity). Don agreed to try the plan, and after two months, his pain and bleeding were completely eliminated. He thanked me for saving him from the ordeal of surgery.

COMMON CAUSES OF HEMORRHOIDS

According to the National Institutes of Health, an estimated 50% of American adults develop hemorrhoids by age 50. However, when you speak with proctologists (medical doctors who specialize in diseases of the rectum, anus and colon), they will tell you that *everyone* has at least some hemorrhoidal tissue, even though many people don't experience symptoms. Problematic hemorrhoids are found equally in men and women, and the prevalence of this condition peaks between ages 45 and 65.

Hemorrhoids, also known as piles, occur when veins and soft tissue around the anus or lower rectum become swollen and inflamed as a result of pressure from straining or carrying extra body weight and/or irritation due to diet. The most common culprits are constipation (especially when a person strains to pass stools)…obesity (extra body weight bears down on veins in the lower rectum, causing pressure)…and pregnancy/childbirth (the fetus increases pressure on the pelvic and rectal tissues, and hormonal changes make blood vessels more lax). Diarrhea associated with inflammatory bowel diseases, such as Crohn's disease and ulcerative colitis, can cause significant irritation that predisposes sufferers to hemorrhoids.

Hemorrhoids are often the cause of bleeding from the anus. This is due to the rich network of veins in tissues of the rectum and anal canal. Besides pain, other common hemorrhoidal symptoms include itching and burning in the anal area.

Caution: If you experience excessive or recurrent rectal bleeding, discuss it with your doctor. Although hemorrhoids are a common cause of such bleeding, other conditions, such as colon cancer, may trigger it. To determine the cause of rectal bleeding, your doctor may perform a rectal exam and/or order tests, such as flexible sigmoidoscopy or colonoscopy. For both tests, a tube with a fiber-optic light and lens are inserted through the rectum. Flexible sigmoidoscopy examines one-third of the colon. Colonoscopy examines the entire colon.

Internal hemorrhoids are located at the top of the anal canal, where they can be seen only with a special examining scope called an anoscope. They are usually painless, and many people are unaware that they have them unless the piles bleed. Large internal hemorrhoids can protrude outside the anus during a bowel movement. In this case, the stool may be accompanied by mucus and bright red blood, which also may appear on toilet paper and/or can be seen in the toilet bowl.

Hemorrhoids that originate at the lower end of the anal canal near the anus are referred to as external hemorrhoids. They can become quite painful and tender to the touch due to the large number of nerves in the anus. Inflamed external hemorrhoids can turn blue or purple as the veins become engorged with blood. Blood clots are more likely to occur in external hemorrhoids than in internal hemorrhoids. Clots create the sensation of a very painful lump. They're not as dangerous as blood clots in other parts of the circulatory system but still may require medical attention, including surgical removal.

CONVENTIONAL TREATMENT OPTIONS

There are a variety of conventional therapies for hemorrhoids. They include ointments, creams and suppositories, all of which provide temporary relief from rectal pain and itching. Common over-the-counter topical treatments include ointments and suppositories, such as Anusol and Preparation H, as well as Tucks medicated wipes. Stool softeners such as *docusate sodium* (Colace) are commonly recommended. These treatments can provide temporary relief, but they don't address the root causes of hemorrhoids.

Internal hemorrhoids that are confined to the anal canal become a problem if they prolapse and bulge from the anus. If this occurs, they are candidates for several procedures, each of which destroys the affected tissue and leaves a scar at the treatment site. The procedures include *ligation* (putting a rubber band around hemorrhoids so that the tissue dies)…*sclerotherapy* (injecting chemicals into the hemorrhoid, causing shrinkage)…*heat coagulation* (using heat from lasers to destroy hemorrhoidal tissue)…and *cryotherapy* (freezing of hemorrhoidal tissue).

Large hemorrhoids that protrude from the anal canal and/or cause bleeding that is difficult to control are commonly removed by surgery. *Hemorrhoidectomy* involves surgical removal of internal and/or external hemorrhoids from the anal canal by cutting out the hemorrhoidal tissue and stitching the site. Postsurgical pain is a major problem with this procedure, and strong pain medications are required for days to weeks. Patients are also told to sit on a large, soft "donut" to ease pressure after the surgery.

Even so, I remember one patient telling me that his postsurgical rectal pain was so intense that for two days, even with the strongest of painkillers, he lay in his bed, knocking his head against a wall. Patients don't typically return to work for two to four weeks. Other complications may include painful bowel movements, difficulty urinating, hemorrhaging, infection, narrowing of the anus (due to scarring) and bowel incontinence. Obviously, this type of surgery should be used only as a last resort.

AN IMPROVED DIET TO THE RESCUE

Hemorrhoids are yet another result of the typical Western diet. People who live in countries where fiber intake is high, such as Japan, have a very low incidence of hemorrhoids. The problem is that the average American consumes only about 15 g of fiber daily. For efficient bowel movements, a person should consume about 25 g to 30 g of fiber daily.

Insoluble fiber, which is found mainly in whole grains and vegetables, bulks up the stool and allows for better elimination. In addition to increasing your intake of these foods, it is imperative that you drink enough water, which allows for easier bowel movements by preventing dryness and adding weight to stool. If you are prone to constipation, drink 64 ounces of water daily, spread throughout the day. As I have mentioned before, ground flaxseed is an excellent source of insoluble fiber. I recommend using one to two tablespoons daily of ground flaxseed (grind fresh flaxseed in a coffee grinder for five seconds or buy preground flaxseed, known as flaxmeal) on cereal, yogurt, salads, etc. It adds a delicious, nutty flavor. Drink at least 10 ounces of water immediately after consuming flaxseed. As an alternative to flaxseed, people who are prone to hard stools or straining should use one to two tablespoons of flaxseed oil—it lubricates stool. Take flaxseed oil with meals or add it to salads or shakes.

Researchers have confirmed the importance of fiber for the treatment of hemorrhoids. A study published in the *American Journal of Gastroenterology* reviewed seven trials involving a total of 378 patients who received either fiber or a nonfiber placebo over the course of one to 18 months. Compared with people who received a placebo, the fiber group's risk of persistent hemorrhoidal symptoms decreased by 47% and their risk of bleeding decreased by 50%.

Not surprisingly, certain foods can aggravate hemorrhoids. These include coffee and other caffeine-containing products, alcohol, spicy foods and high-sugar products, such as soft drinks and candy. In addition, patients who are prone to repeated hemorrhoidal flare-ups usually do better when they reduce or eliminate their intake of tomatoes, cow's milk, citrus fruit, wheat and peanuts. No one knows exactly why these foods and drinks are problematic, but they most likely cause veins to swell.

SOOTHING SUPPLEMENTS WORK WONDERS

I consistently find the following nutritional supplements to be effective in treating and preventing hemorrhoids. If you have an acute flare-up, I recommend taking the first two or more supplements for quicker healing. After symptoms subside, continue taking them for two months to prevent a recurrence. If your symptoms don't improve after using the first two supplements for 30 days, consider taking the others listed below (individually or in a combination formula) for a more aggressive approach. All of the products are available at health-food stores and some pharmacies.

•**Horse chestnut** improves circulation to the rectal area and reduces swelling of hemorrhoidal tissue. One of the herb's most important active constituents is *aescin*. It is believed to strengthen the vein walls and capillaries—and helps with the functioning of vein valves—so that swelling is less likely to occur. Take 400 mg to 600 mg of horse chestnut three times daily. Choose a product that contains 40 mg to 120 mg of aescin per capsule.

Important: Because horse chestnut may have a mild blood-thinning effect, it should not

be used by anyone taking a blood-thinner, such as *warfarin* (Coumadin).

•**Butcher's broom** is an herb that reduces hemorrhoidal symptoms, such as bleeding and pain. *Ruscogenins,* a primary constituent, are believed to have an anti-inflammatory effect on hemorrhoidal tissue. Take a total daily dose of 200 mg to 300 mg of butcher's broom with 9% to 11% ruscogenins. This supplement is very safe, with only rare reports of nausea.

•**Bilberry,** an herbal supplement that's well known for promoting eye health, also helps hemorrhoids, most likely because it strengthens blood vessel walls and improves circulation. A four-week, double-blind, placebo-controlled study of 40 hemorrhoid patients showed that bilberry significantly reduced hemorrhoidal symptoms. In my practice, I've received good results with virtually all my hemorrhoid patients who try bilberry. I recommend taking 320 mg daily of a 25% *anthocyanoside* extract. Bilberry can be used during flare-ups or on an ongoing basis for prevention.

•**Psyllium seed husks** are used as a supplement to treat constipation. Some people find that taking psyllium capsules is more convenient than adding flaxseed to food. Take 3 g to 4 g of psyllium in capsule form with 8 ounces of water twice daily. People who are prone to digestive upset should start with 1 g and slowly work up to 3 g over a period of three weeks.

Caution: Do not use psyllium within two hours of taking a pharmaceutical medication—it can hinder absorption of the drug.

•**Witch hazel,** an astringent derived from the bark of the witch hazel shrub, works well as a topical treatment to soothe inflamed, bleeding hemorrhoids. It's available in cream and liquid forms. Use a cotton ball to dab it on the hemorrhoid three or four times daily and after bowel movements during flare-ups.

A SECRET HEMORRHOID CURE

For nearly three decades, Steve Gardner, ND, DC, has been the nation's foremost expert in natural hemorrhoid therapies. Dr. Gardner holds degrees in naturopathic medicine and chiropractic. He is an assistant professor at the National College of Naturopathic Medicine in Portland, Oregon, teaching proctology. Patients with acute and chronic hemorrhoid problems come to his clinic near Portland from all over the world to benefit from his noninvasive therapy for internal and external hemorrhoids.

More than a decade ago, I treated patients with him at his clinic. Many had experienced the horrors of hemorrhoid surgery and were unwilling to go through such an ordeal again. Many patients told me of the seemingly miraculous relief they had experienced with Dr. Gardner's therapy.

Dr. Gardner and a limited number of doctors (mostly naturopathic and chiropractic physicians) use a procedure known as the Keesey Technique. Wilbur Keesey, MD, developed this technique in the 1930s and never reported a severe complication in more than 700 individual treatments. (Dr. Gardner has performed this therapy several thousand times.) The technique is not FDA approved, but it has a strong history of clinical efficacy.

During this outpatient procedure, known as *hemorrhoidolysis,* the doctor touches the protruding hemorrhoids with an electrode that conducts a galvanic (electrical) current. This type of current causes the hemorrhoids to shrink. The Keesey Technique leads to only slight discomfort, hemorrhage rarely occurs and infection is rare. Because hemorrhoidal tissue is shrunk through the use of this technique, hemorrhoid recurrence is uncommon. There is no loss of time from work, no special preoperative treatment is required, and the procedure costs about $1,500 to $2,000 less than hemorrhoid surgery.

For patients with moderate to severe hemorrhoids, Dr. Gardner usually gives a series of six to 10 treatments with one to two treatments a week. Patients typically have one or two more treatments three months later as a routine follow-up. The cost is $95 per treatment. Dr. Gardner states that about half of his patients' health insurers cover the treatments.

The Keesey Technique offers relief even for people who have extensive hemorrhoidal swelling that does not respond to dietary changes, supplement use and regular exercise. Dr. Gardner has found that less than 5% of the patients he treats require a referral for surgery.

To locate a physician who uses the Keesey Technique, contact the American Association of Naturopathic Physicians, 866-538-2267, *www. naturopathic.org.* Or see Dr. Gardner or one of his colleagues at his Sandy Boulevard Hemorrhoid Clinic East in Milwaukie, Oregon, 503-786-7272 or 888-664-6662, *www.hemorrhoid help.com.*

Chronic Viral Infection

Viruses take many forms—some much more pernicious—and now I want to add even more weapons to your antivirus arsenal. Let me tell you about Michael, a 16-year-old from Georgia.

Michael developed an illness that kept him out of school for six weeks. It had begun with flulike symptoms. Six weeks later, he still had muscle aches and pains, head congestion, relentless fatigue and chills. To top it off, reflux—in which stomach acid backflows into the esophagus—continued to plague him. Tests by his doctors showed that Michael had had mononucleosis in the past, but there were no current signs of infection. Since he had been healthy before this, his father was frustrated by the lack of treatment options offered by his hometown doctors, so he scheduled a phone conference with me.

READING THE BATTLE SCARS

Blood tests ordered by Michael's previous doctors had shown that he had a low level of a certain kind of white blood cells called lymphocytes. This finding, combined with his particular symptoms, suggested to me that his *lymphocytes* were burned out from fighting an infection. It was evident that Michael had a lingering viral infection that his immune system could not easily fight off.

Michael's father had already given him the immune system–boosting supplements that I usually recommend. These include the herbs echinacea and lomatium, which stimulate white blood cell activity…vitamin C, which also enhances white blood cell activity and activates *interferon,* an antiviral substance in the body…and other herbal combinations of immune boosters. Although these types of supplements usually work well

133

to destroy a virus, it was clear that we needed a different approach in Michael's case.

THE HEALING PROCESS

In addition to the remedies Michael was taking, I asked him to add homeopathic gelsemium. This remedy, made using a highly diluted plant extract, is excellent for viral infections that cause muscle aches, fatigue and chills. He took two 30C-strength pellets two times daily. I also suggested 40 drops a day of an herbal immune builder known as *maitake*. I chose this mushroom extract because Michael's illness had become chronic. Maitake is a good choice for long-term immune enhancement because it maintains a constant activation of immune cells.

When I spoke with Michael's father two weeks later, his son's energy had greatly improved, the reflux was gone and his muscles ached only at the end of the day. I recommended that Michael continue taking the antiviral therapies and maitake. I also suggested that he avoid simple sugars, such as those found in juice, white bread and candy, because they suppress white blood cell activity. I suggested that he eat soups, stews and steamed vegetables, which are easy to digest, to continue building his energy. Because the adrenal glands of people with chronic infections often become fatigued, compromising a healthy immune response, I added a prescription supplement to Michael's regimen to support these glands. In two more weeks, Michael was able to return to school. He is still doing well a year later.

Fight Osteoporosis The Natural Way— Simple Steps... For Women and Men

Misconceptions abound when it comes to osteoporosis, a dreaded disease that's marked by porous, brittle bones and hunched backs. Most people think of osteoporosis as a women's disease, but it's more than that. While 8 million American women have been diagnosed with osteoporosis, more than 2 million men also are affected by it.

OSTEOPOROSIS: A SILENT PROBLEM

Osteoporosis can develop because, starting at about age 35, our bone cells do not make new bone as fast as it is broken down. Our bones become more frail and fracture more easily. Fractures, especially of the hip, spine and wrist, are more likely to occur, even without trauma. Osteoporosis has no symptoms until a bone is fractured. Many people go for decades without a diagnosis of osteoporosis—until they fall and an X-ray reveals porous bones.

Bone density can be measured with a dual-energy X-ray absorptiometry (DEXA) scan, but many people don't get this test. I recommend a baseline DEXA scan by age 50, and if results are normal, follow-ups every three to five years.

The most worrisome risk for a person with osteoporosis is a hip fracture. According to the National Osteoporosis Foundation (*www.nof.org*), an average of 24% of hip-fracture patients age 50 or older die in the year following their fractures, often as a result of long-term immobilization that leads to blood clots or infection. Six months after a hip fracture, only 15% of patients can walk unaided across a room.

Virtually every person with osteoporosis who has come to my clinic is confused about the best way to promote bone health. Conventional doctors typically prescribe osteoporosis medication, such as *alendronate* (Fosamax) and *ibandronate* (Boniva). However, these drugs can cause side effects, such as digestive upset and blood clots, and they don't address the underlying nutritional deficiencies that promote bone loss.

The natural protocol I recommend includes a healthful diet (rich in vegetables, fruit and fish and low in refined-sugar products and red meat)...weight-bearing exercise (such as walking and stair-climbing)...and good hormone balance (deficiencies of some hormones, such as testosterone, accelerate bone loss). I also suggest certain bone-protecting supplements.

Caution: People with kidney disease should not take supplements without consulting a doctor. With kidney disease, the kidneys cannot process high doses of nutrients.

My recommendations for women and men: To help prevent osteoporosis, take the first three supplements listed below. If you have osteoporosis or osteopenia (mild bone loss that can be diagnosed with a DEXA scan), take the first three supplements listed and as many of the others as you're willing to try, in the dosages recommended...

SUPER TRIO PREVENTS AND TREATS OSTEOPOROSIS

•**Calcium is the most prevalent mineral in bone tissue.** Taking supplements helps prevent a deficiency. Most studies have found that calcium slows bone loss but does not increase bone density when used alone. Women with osteoporosis should take 500 mg of calcium twice daily with meals. It should be a well-absorbed form, such as citrate, citrate-malate, amino acid chelate or hydroxyapatite. To boost absorption, take no more than 500 mg per dose. Calcium carbonate, which is widely used, is *not* well-absorbed. For osteoporosis prevention, men and women, as well as boys and girls starting at age 13, should take 500 mg daily.

Calcium supplementation for men with osteoporosis is more complicated. Some recent research has identified a link between high calcium intake (from dairy products) and increased prostate cancer risk. A meta-analysis in the *Journal of the National Cancer Institute* that reviewed 12 studies on this association concluded, "High intake of dairy products and calcium may be associated with an increased risk for prostate cancer, although the increase appears to be small." A recent study found that calcium intake exceeding 1,500 mg a day (from food and supplements) may be associated with a higher risk of advanced, and potentially fatal, prostate cancer. The saturated fat in dairy products may raise prostate cancer risk.

Until there is more definitive information, I recommend that men who have osteoporosis, regardless of whether they have eliminated calcium-rich foods from their diets, take no more than a 500-mg calcium supplement daily. Men with prostate cancer should consult their doctors before using calcium supplements.

•**Vitamin D** promotes absorption of calcium. Deficiencies of this vitamin are more common in Americans over age 50 than in younger adults. Sun exposure prompts the body to produce vitamin D, and the kidneys help convert it to its active form. As we age, our skin cannot synthesize vitamin D as effectively from sunlight,

and our kidneys become less efficient. People with darker skin, those with digestive problems (due to malabsorption conditions, such as Crohn's disease) and those with limited exposure to sunlight are also at greater risk for vitamin D deficiency. Preliminary studies indicate that an inadequate intake of vitamin D is associated with an increased risk of fractures.

For the prevention of osteoporosis, I recommend 600 IU to 800 IU of vitamin D daily. People with osteoporosis should take 800 IU to 1,200 IU daily. Vitamin D is fat soluble, meaning it is better absorbed when taken with meals (containing small amounts of fat).

For many patients with low vitamin D levels, I recommend 2,000 IU of vitamin D daily. To ensure that vitamin D levels are optimal, I monitor blood levels once or twice a year. Overdosing can lead to heart arrhythmia, anorexia, nausea and other ill effects.

•**Magnesium,** an important constituent of bone crystals, is crucial for the proper metabolism of calcium. A deficiency of magnesium impairs bone-building cells known as *osteoblasts*. Like calcium, magnesium requires vitamin D for absorption.

Researchers at Tel Aviv University in Israel looked at the effect of magnesium supplementation on bone density in 31 postmenopausal women with osteoporosis. This two-year, open, controlled trial (both the researchers and patients knew who was receiving the placebo or the supplement) involved giving the participants 250 mg to 750 mg of magnesium daily for six months and 250 mg for another 18 months. Twenty-two patients (71%) experienced a 1% to 8% increase in bone density. The mean bone density of all treated patients increased significantly after one year and remained at that level after two years. Among an additional 23 postmenopausal women not receiving magnesium, mean bone density *decreased* significantly.

For osteoporosis prevention, take 400 mg to 500 mg of magnesium daily...for osteoporosis, take 500 mg to 750 mg daily. In both cases, take in divided doses.

IF YOU HAVE BONE-LOSS DISEASE

•**Vitamin K** has received attention in recent years for its role in treating osteoporosis. It activates *osteocalcin,* a bone protein that regulates calcium metabolism in the bones and helps calcium bind to the tissues that make up the bone. It also has been shown to inhibit inflammatory chemicals that cause bone breakdown.

Studies have shown that low vitamin K intake and blood levels are associated with reduced bone density and fractures in people who have osteoporosis. A recent meta-analysis published in the American Medical Association's *Archives of Internal Medicine* found that vitamin K supplements were associated with a consistent reduction in all types of fractures. Leafy, green vegetables, such as spinach, kale, collard greens and broccoli, are the best sources of vitamin K, yet many people do not consume these vitamin K–rich foods on a regular basis. High-dose vitamin K (above 2 mg) should be used only under the supervision of a doctor, because excess vitamin K may increase blood clotting. Vitamin K supplements should not be used by people who take blood-thinning medication, such as *warfarin* (Coumadin) or *heparin,* or by pregnant women or nursing mothers. I typically recommend 2 mg to 10 mg daily of vitamin K for people who have osteoporosis to help increase their bone density.

•**Essential fatty acids** (EFAs) have been shown to improve bone density in older women and are believed also to promote bone health in men. Many researchers theorize that osteoporosis develops because of chronic inflammation of bone tissue (due to stress, toxins, poor diet and infection). EFAs, especially those found in fish oil, reduce inflammation. Some studies show that EFAs also improve calcium absorption. I recommend that people with osteoporosis take fish oil daily (containing about 480 mg of EPA and 320 mg of DHA), along with 3,000 mg of evening primrose oil, which contains inflammation-fighting gamma-linolenic acid (GLA). Because EFAs have a blood-thinning effect, check with your doctor if you are taking a blood thinner.

•**Strontium** is a mineral that does not get much attention, because it is not regarded as essential for the human body. However, 99% of the total amount of strontium found in the body is located in the teeth and bones. Supplemental strontium is not the radioactive type that you may have heard about in relation to nuclear facilities.

Strontium is a valuable mineral for people with osteoporosis, and I often recommend it.

A clinical trial in the *New England Journal of Medicine* found that strontium prevents vertebral fractures and increases bone density. The most common supplemental forms are strontium chloride and strontium citrate. I suggest a supplement that contains 680 mg of elemental strontium daily (similar to the dose used in most studies). Because calcium inhibits strontium absorption, strontium should be taken at least four hours before or after calcium is taken. Strontium should not be taken by pregnant women and nursing mothers. It is not available at most health-food stores, but you can buy it from Vitacost (800-381-0759, *www.vitacost.com*). A one-month supply costs about $20.

•**Soy,** as a supplement and/or food, has been shown in several studies to improve bone density. Soy contains *isoflavones,* estrogen-like constituents that support bone mass and relieve menopausal symptoms in women. Women and men with osteoporosis or osteopenia should take 125 mg of soy isoflavones daily in soy protein powder or supplement form and consume three to five servings of soy foods weekly. (One serving equals one-half cup of tofu…one-half cup of soy beans…or one cup of soy milk.)

Caution: Soy supplements are not well studied in women who have had breast cancer, so they should avoid supplements and nonfermented soy products.

•**Vitamin C** is required for the production of the protein *collagen,* a component of bone tissue. I recommend that people with osteoporosis take 1,000 mg twice daily. Reduce the dosage if loose stools develop.

•**Silicon** is a trace mineral required for bone formation. I recommend 2 mg to 5 mg daily.

BEST OSTEOPOROSIS FORMULAS

These products contain all the vitamins and minerals described in this article, in the therapeutic doses used for osteoporosis treatment…

•**Bone Up** by Jarrow. To find an on-line retailer, call 800-726-0886 or go to *www.jarrow.com.*

•**Osteoprime** by Enzymatic Therapy. To find a retailer, call 800-783-2286 or go to *www. enzy.com.*

.Pro Bone by Ortho Molecular Products is available from health-care professionals, including naturopaths, holistic MDs, chiropractors, nutritionists and acupuncturists. If you cannot locate a health-care professional in your area who sells the formula, it is available from my clinic at 858-450-7120, *www.lajollawholehealth.com.*

Calcium and Kidney Stones

Recently, one of my readers passed a very small kidney stone. Her doctor took her completely off calcium. She began developing a curved spine. Was it necessary to drop the calcium?

I suggested other options. A kidney stone is a small, hard mass made up of crystals. When a kidney stone breaks loose and begins to make its way from your kidneys to your bladder through the connecting tube (ureter), it can cause severe back pain that may radiate to the groin area.

There are different types of kidney stones—80% of them are composed of calcium salts. People with a history of kidney stones may need to avoid calcium supplements. Some people absorb calcium more readily than others. Those who are calcium "hyperabsorbers" are at greatest risk. I told my reader that her doctor can test her calcium absorption with a 24-hour urinary calcium test. If the urine test does not show high levels of calcium, she could probably take a supplement under her doctor's supervision.

Interestingly, calcium citrate (calcium bound to citric acid) actually may prevent some kidney stones. It's not clear why calcium citrate, as opposed to another type of calcium supplement, does this, but it may be its acidic nature. It is thought that citrate binds with calcium in the urine, reducing the amount of calcium available to form calcium oxalate stones. (*Oxalate,* a compound found in spinach, chocolate, tea and other foods, forms an insoluble substance with calcium to develop this most common type of kidney stone.) Calcium citrate is also thought to prevent tiny calcium oxalate crystals from growing and forming into larger stones—and it makes

the urine less acidic, which inhibits development of both calcium oxalate and uric acid stones.

With normal calcium testing, up to 800 mg of calcium citrate can be taken in divided doses daily with meals. Also, studies show that supplementation with 500 mg of magnesium and 100 mg of vitamin B-6 daily can significantly decrease the recurrence of kidney stones. In addition, red meat consumption should be reduced. Red meat increases urinary calcium. Drink 64 ounces of water daily to flush calcium oxalate crystals out of the body.

Castor Oil— Quick Fix for Constipation?

One of my readers informed me that he had begun taking castor oil for his chronic constipation. He asked me if it was harmful.

Castor oil comes from the seeds of the castor bean and has long been used to treat constipation. It aids elimination by preventing absorption of liquids from the intestinal tract, but prolonged use can lead to a depletion of minerals, especially potassium. It should be used as a laxative only for a few days. Repeated use contributes to a "lazy" digestive tract, which can worsen constipation in the long run.

If constipation is a frequent problem for you, consult your doctor to make sure that there is no medical cause, such as thyroid disease or a tumor in the digestive tract. Also, I have found that taking two tablespoons of ground flaxseed with 10 ounces of water each morning helps many patients. Flaxseed has other benefits, too—it's rich in healthful omega-3 fatty acids and has cancer-preventing properties. In addition, be sure to drink water throughout the day—ideally one-half ounce per pound of body weight up to 64 ounces a day. Regular exercise also encourages bowel regularity.

SPECIAL REPORT #7:

How to Spot Health Problems Early by Reading Your Body's Hidden Signals

How to Spot Health Problems Early by Reading Your Body's Hidden Signals

Head-to-Toe Diagnostic Clues—Part 1

Stand in front of a mirror and stick out your tongue. Is your tongue's surface smooth or cracked? Stroke your fingers across the back of your upper arm. Do you feel tiny bumps on the skin? You may never have noticed—but to a holistic doctor, such small physical signs provide clues to your health. Close observation gives me a sense of a patient's problem even before I hear about symptoms or see lab test results—giving us a head start on healing.

WHAT YOUR HAIR AND FACE REVEAL ABOUT YOUR HEALTH

In a two-part feature, I'll take you on a top-to-bottom tour of the body, describing subtle signs that suggest health problems and outlining treatments. Unless noted, all products are sold at health-food stores or pharmacies and are safe for everyone (but if you take medication, check with your doctor before using them). In cases where my advice may differ from the instructions on product labels, I have recommended dosages. We'll cover the hair and face and the rest of the body (including the arm and its mysterious bumps).

HAIR'S HEALTH CLUES

•**Brittle hair.** Hair that breaks easily and has split ends may signal nutritional deficiencies. I suggest taking supplements of the mineral *silicon* at 5 mg daily...the sulfur compound *methylsulfonylmethane* (MSM) at 3,000 mg daily...and a vitamin B complex at 50 mg twice daily. Essential fatty acids (EFAs) also help, so take fish oil supplements with 500 mg to 1,000 mg of combined *eicosapentaenoic acid* (EPA) and *docosahexaenoic acid* (DHA), or two tablespoons daily of flaxseed oil, perilla oil or hemp seed oil.

Mark A. Stengler, ND, naturopathic physician in private practice, La Jolla, California...adjunct associate clinical professor at the National College of Natural Medicine, Portland, Oregon...author of many books, including *The Natural Physician's Healing Therapies* and coauthor of *Prescription for Natural Cures* (both from Bottom Line Books)...and author of the *Bottom Line/Natural Healing* newsletter.

Helpful: Shampoo enriched with vitamin B-7 (*biotin*), such as Natural Biotin Hair Fortifying Shampoo (Jason Natural Products, 877-527-6601, *www.jason-natural.com*).

•**Hair loss.** It's often blamed on genes, but for some men and most women, hair loss is actually due to excess *cortisol* (a stress hormone) or testosterone…or deficiencies of estrogen, progesterone or thyroid hormone. Low thyroid hormone also causes partial loss of the eyebrows. Such imbalances are associated with poor diet, stress, exposure to toxins or (for women) pregnancy or menopause. Hormone imbalances can be confirmed with saliva, urine and/or blood testing.

Mild cases of hair loss can be corrected in men and women with natural over-the-counter (OTC) remedies. *Try…*

•The herbs saw palmetto (for men) or chasteberry (for women).

•A cream containing progesterone (for women). Use under the supervision of a doctor—excessive dosages may cause irregular menstrual cycles.

If hair loss occurs at a time of high stress, also take oral supplements of…

•The herb ashwagandha (in extract form).

•An herbal relaxation formula with passionflower, oat straw and/or valerian root.

If these remedies don't halt hair loss within six weeks, you may have a severe hormone imbalance. Talk to your doctor about bioidentical prescription hormone therapy.

•**Sensitive scalp.** When patients report that it hurts to comb their hair, I suspect a deficiency of nutrients involved with nerve function.

Solution: Daily supplements of vitamin D at 800 international units (IU) to 2,000 IU, plus 500 mg of magnesium in divided doses. Scalp pain also can be due to a sensitivity to shampoos or styling products. Switch to more natural hair products, available at health-food stores.

•**Dandruff.** It doesn't take a doctor to spot telltale flakes, but few people realize that dandruff often stems from nutritional deficiencies. Take a vitamin B complex at 50 mg twice daily…a multivitamin that includes 200 micrograms (mcg) of the mineral selenium…and EFAs, such as fish oil or flaxseed, perilla or hemp seed oil.

Dandruff also may be linked to low stomach acid, which impedes nutrient absorption.

Helpful: OTC tablets of *betaine hydrochloride* (which mimics stomach acid), at 500 mg to 700 mg three times daily with meals, plus the herbs gentian root and dandelion root, which stimulate stomach acid production. (Do not use these if you have an ulcer.)

SECRETS SEEN IN THE EYES

•**Bloodshot eyes.** Persistent eye redness without nasal congestion suggests a food sensitivity, typically to dairy products, soy, sugar, wheat or gluten (a sticky protein found in wheat, rye and barley). To identify triggers, eliminate suspected foods from your diet, one by one, for several weeks to see if symptoms improve.

Unique diagnostic tool: Noninvasive *electrodermal testing*, which measures the body's electrical response—at acupuncture points and energy-flow meridians—to the foods being tested. (This test is available from holistic physicians and chiropractors.) Also, blood testing can measure the body's production of antibodies in response to various foods. Foods that trigger reactions can be avoided…or a desensitization program that involves exposure to small but steadily increasing amounts of the allergen can "teach" the immune system to stop overreacting.

•**Dark circles.** This classic sign of sleep deprivation also can indicate food allergies. Less often, dark circles suggest that the liver is not effectively removing toxins from the body. To improve liver function, eat carrots and beets or drink their juices…and take daily supplements of *chlorella* (a type of algae), plus the herbs milk thistle, dandelion root and wheatgrass.

•**Pale inner eyelids.** When I gently pull down a patient's lower eyelid, I hope to see a healthy pink-red color. A pale eyelid interior suggests iron-deficiency anemia—especially if the patient has bleeding hemorrhoids…has a heavy menstrual flow…or is a vegan (one who eats no meat, fish, dairy foods, eggs or honey). If blood tests confirm an iron deficiency, I prescribe 100 mg to 200 mg of chelated iron daily, to be taken only until test results return to normal.

EAR EXAM

•**Earwax.** Excessive buildup often signals a food sensitivity or an EFA deficiency. To remove earwax, place two drops of warm (not hot) olive oil in the affected ear…leave in for one hour (lie on your side, ear up)…then rinse in the shower or bathtub. Repeat as necessary. OTC earwax removal products with peroxide can be used in a similar manner.

•**Popping noises.** Often due to chronic *serous otitis media* (fluid behind the eardrum), these noises may be caused by an EFA deficiency or food sensitivities.

Helpful: A naturopathic or osteopathic doctor or a chiropractor can gently manipulate the head and neck to release trapped fluid.

WHAT I KNOW FROM A NOSE

•**Runny nose.** When red eyes accompany a runny nose, I suspect an environmental allergy —to pollen or dust mites, for example. For relief, take supplements of stinging nettle leaf and *quercetin* (an anti-inflammatory plant compound)… and rinse eyes twice daily with one ounce of saline solution mixed with five drops of the herb *eyebright* in tincture form.

•**Red nose.** Flushing on the nose and cheeks that's accompanied by red bumps may look like pimples, but it could be due to the inflammatory skin disease *rosacea*. Its cause is unknown, though there may be an underlying vascular problem. A bacterial infection called *Helicobacter pylori* (which also causes stomach ulcers) may be associated with rosacea, too. Such an infection can be diagnosed with a blood test and treated with antibiotics or oral supplements of the amino acid *zinc carnosine*…the herbal preparation *mastic gum*…and/or betaine hydrochloride. Since bacteria on the skin may exacerbate problems, use a topical cream with the compound alpha lipoic acid. Too much estrogen and/or too little progesterone also may contribute to rosacea.

Helpful: Hormone-balancing progesterone capsules or cream (for women)…or the herb burdock root in capsule form, at 500 mg three times daily (for men and women).

WHAT A MOUTH TELLS ME

•**Swollen gums.** These usually indicate poor dental hygiene, but they also can suggest a deficiency of vitamin C or *flavonoids* (healthful plant pigments), especially if the patient bruises easily. Try 1,000 mg of vitamin C twice daily…plus 300 mg of grape seed extract daily. In a vegetarian or a person who takes cholesterol-lowering statin drugs, swollen gums suggest a deficiency of the naturally occurring nutrient coenzyme Q10 (CoQ10), needed for basic cell function.

Helpful: 100 mg to 200 mg of CoQ10 daily.

•**Pale or swollen tongue.** A light red tongue is a sign of good health, but a pale pink tongue may indicate iron deficiency. A swollen, smooth, sore tongue suggests a deficiency of B vitamins. Blood tests can confirm deficiencies, and supplements or injections can correct the problem.

•**White tongue coating.** A thin coating is normal, but a thick white coating suggests a *Candida albicans* yeast infection—either limited to the mouth or reflecting an overgrowth of yeast in the digestive tract. It is common with long-term use of antibiotics. Restrict simple sugars…eat yogurt with live cultures…take antifungal herbs, such as oregano oil…and take probiotics, such as *Lactobacillus acidophilus* and *bifidobacterium*, to restore beneficial bacteria to the digestive tract.

•**Rough tongue.** Grooves in the middle of the tongue plus a sticky coating of mucus are associated with chronic digestive problems, such as irritable bowel syndrome (IBS) or ulcerative colitis. Scalloped indentations on the sides of the tongue suggest liver or gallbladder problems.

Solutions: A more healthful diet…digestive enzyme supplements, such as Enzymedica Digest Gold (888-918-1118, *www.enzymedica.com*), taken with meals…herbs to aid digestion, including ginger and gentian root…and/or herbs that support liver and gallbladder function, such as milk thistle, turmeric, artichoke and dandelion.

•**Splotchy tongue.** Small bumps called *papillae* normally cover the tongue's upper surface. Smooth, sensitive splotches amidst the bumpiness result from the loss of papillae on certain areas, creating a "geographic tongue."

Likely cause: Vitamin B deficiency. Take 50 mg of a vitamin B complex twice daily.

Also try: The homeopathic remedy *Taraxacum* (derived from dandelion root). Take two pellets of a 30C potency twice daily for two weeks.

143

CHEEK CHECKUP

•**Sunken cheeks.** Few American doctors realize that hollow cheeks can indicate a deficiency of cortisol or growth hormone. Saliva or blood testing can identify the problem, which then can be treated with hormone therapy, if necessary.

•**Puffy cheeks.** I can tell whether a woman takes birth control pills because her puffy cheeks are a tip-off. Daily supplements of 50 mg of vitamin B-6 and 500 mg of magnesium help the liver to process the estrogen from the pills, reducing water retention.

Now that you know what to watch for, give your head a good look. If you notice any of the signs above, talk to your doctor—who will applaud your diagnostic skills.

Head-to-Toe Diagnostic Clues—Part 2

Stroke your fingers across the back of your upper arm. Do you feel tiny bumps on the skin? When I asked this earlier, I left readers wondering—because Part 1 of this two-part feature discussed what the face and hair reveal about health. In Part 2, I'll review the rest of the body—and share the secret behind those tiny bumps, plus many other subtle health clues.

Unless noted, all treatments below are safe for everyone. Supplements are sold at health-food stores.

NEWS FROM THE NECK

•**Bowtie-shaped bump.** This distinctive swelling at the base of the throat is a *goiter,* or enlarged thyroid gland, due to a deficiency of iodine. The thyroid gland needs iodine to manufacture thyroid hormone. Deficiencies are common in people who avoid salt.

Solution: Eat iodine-rich sea vegetables, strawberries, eggs and dairy foods (in moderation)…take 150 micrograms (mcg) to 300 mcg of iodine daily in capsule form…and consult an endocrinologist.

•**Stiff neck.** Tight muscles or restriction of the neck vertebrae can result from poor posture or sleeping with a pillow that is too soft or too hard.

Recommended: Massage and/or acupuncture, particularly if you also have headaches or neck pain…a cervical pillow that fits the neck's natural curve…and the muscle-relaxing mineral magnesium (250 mg twice daily), taken with calcium (500 mg twice daily) for optimal effect, until stiffness is gone.

Warning: A stiff neck along with a fever and severe headache may indicate meningitis, a serious infection that requires emergency care.

WHAT THE TORSO TELLS ME

•**Sagging breasts.** In a woman, droopy breasts may simply be her natural shape—or may indicate a deficiency of the hormones estrogen and/or progesterone, particularly if accompanied by hot flashes and overall loss of skin elasticity. If saliva and/or blood tests confirm a deficiency, hormone replacement therapy (HRT) may be appropriate.

Flabby breast tissue is not uncommon in overweight men because fat cells produce estrogen, a hormone that contributes to breast enlargement. A diet rich in cruciferous vegetables (broccoli, cauliflower, collard greens, cabbage), plus two tablespoons of ground flaxseeds daily (taken with 10 ounces of water), help the liver to break down excess estrogen—and also provide a good start on a sensible weight-loss plan.

•**Apple-shaped abdomen.** A person who is as big or bigger around the waist as around the hips may have *insulin resistance*—in which the body's cells don't readily accept the glucose-transporting hormone insulin, so the pancreas produces more insulin to compensate. This leads to an accumulation of fat around the waist. Insulin resistance is a risk factor for diabetes. Excessive insulin also contributes to inflammation—which sets the stage for cardiovascular disease, Alzheimer's disease, arthritis and cancer.

For a rotund patient, I recommend regular exercise and a diet high in fiber and low in refined carbohydrates. Supplements of a fat called *conjugated linoleic acid* (CLA) at 1,000 mg three times daily can aid weight loss and promote the cells' proper use of insulin. Slimaluma, a plant extract (taken at 500 mg, one hour before breakfast and dinner), curbs appetite and reduces abdominal fat. I also test levels of *dehydroepiandrosterone* (DHEA), since supplementation of this hormone in people who have low levels can reduce belly fat and improve insulin resistance.

CLUES IN THE SKIN

.Hairless skin. Sparse body hair in men and women suggests a deficiency of the hormones testosterone and/or DHEA, which can increase the risk for depression, fatigue, poor memory, low libido, osteoporosis and heart disease. If tests confirm the diagnosis, prescription testosterone HRT and/or nonprescription DHEA oral supplements (best used under a doctor's supervision) may be warranted.

.Skin tags. These small, soft, protruding bumps are connected to the skin by a narrow stalk of tissue. They are usually benign and painless but can become irritated. Skin tags are most common on the eyelids, neck, armpits, upper chest and groin...tend to appear in middle age... and are more common in women. Growths can be removed surgically, electrically (cautery) or by freezing (cryotherapy), but they may grow back. The cause of skin tags is unknown, but natural remedies may halt the spread and prevent recurrence. Take daily supplements of biotin (300 mcg)...chromium (200 mcg to 400 mcg)...alpha lipoic acid (300 mg)...and cinnamon extract (500 mg). Also try homeopathic Thuja occidentalis, at two pellets of a 30C potency twice daily for a month.

SECRETS HELD IN THE HANDS & ARMS

.Weak pulse at the wrist. Every doctor checks a patient's pulse, looking for a steady rate of 60 to 80 beats per minute. However, I like to employ some of my Chinese medicine training by evaluating more subtle signs. For example, a very strong pulse can indicate stress, while a weak pulse that is hard to detect suggests that the heart is not contracting as forcefully as it should or that certain organs are not functioning well. A complete pulse diagnosis can be made by a practitioner of Oriental medicine. For a referral, contact the American Association of Acupuncture and Oriental Medicine (866-455-7999, *www.aaaomonline.org*).

.Abnormal fingernails. Spoon-shaped nails or pale nail beds that do not quickly return to their normal color after being pressed suggest iron-deficiency anemia...ridges can indicate infection or low thyroid function...white spots mean a zinc deficiency...and brittle nails signal a deficiency of protein, essential fatty acids, calcium and/or silicon. Nail abnormalities also result from reduced stomach acid, which leads to poor nutrient absorption.

Solution: In addition to a daily multivitamin, take two capsules (with each meal) of *betaine hydrochloride*, a beet extract that increases stomach acid...or a full-spectrum digestive enzyme, which improves nutrient absorption.

LESSONS FROM THE LEGS & FEET

.Stiff knees. A stiff-legged gait and aching knees can signal *osteoarthritis*, a degeneration of cartilage (tough, elastic tissue that allows bones to slide smoothly over one another). Its causes include previous injuries, inflammatory disease and nutritional deficiencies. To lubricate joints and help repair cartilage, take daily glucosamine (1,500 mg)...chondroitin (1,200 mg)...combined *eicosapentaenoic acid* and *docosahexaenoic acid* (1,000 mg)...and *hyaluronic acid* (200 mg in two divided doses).

.Inward- or outward-rolling feet. I watch patients walk, looking for pronation—a biomechanical problem common among the flat-footed, in which the feet tilt inward—or supination, in which the feet roll outward. Either condition can lead to pain in the feet, knees, hips and lower back. A chiropractor or podiatrist can provide supportive custom-made orthotic shoe inserts that promote proper foot alignment.

Helpful: Exercise the muscles of the arch by picking up marbles with your toes.

THE ANSWER YOU'VE BEEN WAITING FOR...

Those itty-bitty, not-so-pretty bumps on the back of the arms are *follicular hyperkeratosis* and usually signal a vitamin A deficiency. Take 5,000 international units (IU)—the upper limit for pregnant women—to 10,000 IU of vitamin A daily until bumps clear up, typically four to six weeks. Thereafter, to prevent a recurrence, take a daily multivitamin that contains at least 2,500 IU of vitamin A or beta-carotene (which the body converts into vitamin A) and eat beta-carotene–rich foods, such as dark green and orange-yellow vegetables.

Excessive Earwax

Earwax eliminates dirt and dead skin from the ear canal. An overabundance of earwax usually is an indication of a chronic sensitivity—either to a food or to something in the environment. Effects from common environmental causes, such as mold, dust and pollen, can be reduced by taking fish oil (1,000 mg daily of combined EPA and DHA), vitamin C (2,000 mg to 3,000 mg) and quercetin (500 mg twice daily). These supplements reduce the response of *histamine*, a chemical produced in the body that triggers allergy symptoms, including the production of earwax.

Common food sensitivities that often contribute to excessive earwax include cow's milk, wheat, soy and sugar. You can try an elimination diet—by avoiding one or more of these foods for two to three weeks—and see if the earwax production lessens.

If these supplements don't help, you should make an appointment with a holistic physician. To find one in your area, contact the American College for Advancement in Medicine (800-532-3688, *www.acam.org*).

The Dangers of Diabetes

More Americans than ever before have *diabetes mellitus*, a disorder characterized by elevated levels of blood sugar (glucose). About 21 million Americans (approximately 7% of the US population) are afflicted with the disease, according to the National Institutes of Health. More than six million of these people don't even realize that they have it.

But that's not all. A staggering 41 million Americans show early signs of diabetes ("prediabetes") but don't know that they are at risk of developing the full-blown disease. This alarming trend is due, in part, to the ever-increasing number of Americans who are overweight, which sharply increases diabetes risk.

If you have been gaining weight, eating a lot of high-fat and high-sugar foods and/or not getting much exercise, I'm afraid that you're already in danger of getting diabetes.

Even though this is a frightening scenario, there is some good news. If you identify the warning signs early enough, you can prevent diabetes from developing. If you already have diabetes, proper monitoring and healthful eating can help you control your glucose levels and avoid many of the disease's serious complications, such as heart failure, stroke, kidney failure, eye disease, nerve damage and/or amputation, due to poor circulation caused by plaque buildup.

WHAT IS DIABETES?

Whenever we eat or drink, the food or liquid we ingest is broken down into nutrients that our bodies need to function. Glucose (a simple sugar that acts as the main energy source for our bodies) is one of the key nutrients. When glucose is absorbed into the bloodstream, it stimulates the pancreas to produce *insulin*. This hormone transports glucose into our body's cells, where it is then converted to energy for immediate or later use.

There are two main types of diabetes...

•**Type 1** (formerly known as juvenile-onset) diabetes affects only about 10% of people with diabetes. Although the disorder usually develops in childhood or early adulthood (before age 30), an increasing number of adults are now being affected.

Researchers theorize that the increasing incidence of obesity in adults may accelerate the autoimmune destruction that characterizes type 1 diabetes—specifically, the body's immune system attacks and destroys the insulin-producing cell destroys the insulin-producing cells of the pancreas.

People with type 1 diabetes need frequent doses of insulin, which is typically delivered by injection with thin needles, a pen that contains an insulin-filled cartridge or a small special "pump" that delivers a continuous dose of insulin. Earlier this year, the FDA approved a new inhaled form of insulin.

•**Type 2** (once known as adult-onset) diabetes affects 90% of people who suffer from the disease. Most cases occur during adulthood, and risk increases with age. In recent years, many overweight children and teenagers have been diagnosed with type 2 diabetes.

In type 2 diabetes, the pancreas produces insulin (often more than the usual amounts), but fat and tissue cells are "resistant," preventing the hormone from doing what it's supposed to do—which is to "unlock" cells so that blood glucose can enter.

Your risk of type 2 diabetes increases significantly if you eat a lot of foods that are high in simple carbohydrates (which are rapidly transformed into sugar) and foods that are low in dietary fiber (needed to slow the absorption of sugars from the food we eat and digest). Also, people who don't get much exercise are more likely to develop type 2 diabetes because of the insulin resistance that results from weight gain and an imbalance of stress hormones.

In addition to obesity, risk factors for type 2 diabetes include a family history of the disease (especially in parents or siblings)...apple-shaped body type...high blood pressure...high cholesterol...or, among women, a history of diabetes during pregnancy ("gestational diabetes," which usually disappears after delivery). People with type 2 diabetes who have difficulty controlling their glucose levels may require oral medication, such as *glucophage* (Metformin), and/or insulin injections.

HEADING OFF DIABETES

Prediabetes affects 40% of Americans between the ages of 40 and 74. In these people, blood glucose levels are elevated but not enough to be considered type 2 diabetes. Detecting the telltale signs of prediabetes—which show up in blood tests—helps you prevent the full-blown disease. Without these measures, there's a good chance that a person diagnosed with prediabetes will develop type 2 diabetes within 10 years.

I advise my patients (and readers) to get yearly blood tests to help identify many early-stage diseases, including diabetes. *Diabetes-related tests should include...*

• **Fasting blood glucose** to determine signs of prediabetes. Before you go to your doctor's office for the test, you will need to fast for at least eight hours. Then blood is drawn and sent to a lab for a measurement of the glucose concentration, which is expressed in milligrams of glucose

per deciliter (mg/dL). A fasting level of 100 mg/dL to 125 mg/dL is considered prediabetes.

Too often, patients who have glucose levels of 100 mg/dL to 115 mg/dL are told by their doctors that they don't have a problem. In my view, a fasting blood glucose level in this range indicates prediabetes. I consider my patients to be free of any immediate risk only if their glucose levels are in the range of 70 mg/dL to 86 mg/dL. If a patient's glucose level is 87 mg/dL to 100 mg/dL, I recommend some of the same strategies that I prescribe for people with prediabetes.

• **Oral glucose tolerance test can be used to check for prediabetes.** After fasting for eight to 12 hours, a blood sample is taken to determine your fasting blood glucose level. Then your doctor will ask you to drink a solution with a high sugar content. After one, two and three hours, your doctor draws a blood sample and checks your glucose reading. A level of 140 mg/dL to 199 mg/dL for any of the readings indicates prediabetes. A reading of 200 mg/dL or above indicates diabetes.

I recommend that doctors also check insulin levels with the blood sample used for the glucose tolerance test. If insulin levels are abnormally high (15 to 20 microunits per milliliter or higher), it's a sign that you are developing insulin resistance—a hallmark of early diabetes.

BETTER DIABETES MONITORING

If you have diabetes, proper monitoring of your condition literally can save your life. Blood sugar levels can change dramatically within a matter of minutes, causing confusion, dizziness, fatigue and, in serious cases, a life-threatening coma. People with diabetes can easily measure their blood sugar levels with a small portable device that analyzes a drop of blood obtained by pricking a fingertip with a lancet. I recommend self-monitoring at least twice daily (upon awakening and 30 to 60 minutes after dinner). In addition, people with diabetes should make regular visits to their primary care doctors, have annual physicals and get yearly eye exams from their ophthalmologists.

Other tests for people with diabetes...

• **Hemoglobin A1C.** This test measures the amount of glucose sticking to the hemoglobin in red blood cells. It can be used as a marker of average blood glucose level over the past two to three months. Studies show that for every percentage point drop in A1C blood levels, risks for circulatory disorders as well as eye, kidney and nerve diseases drop by 40%. Most doctors say that a hemoglobin A1C reading below 7% is acceptable. However, I believe that a reading below 6% is more desirable, because it shows better blood glucose control. People with an A1C reading of 7% or less should have this test twice a year. If your reading is above 8%, you should have it every three months.

•**Oxidative stress analysis.** This test measures the amount of tissue damage, or "oxidative stress," caused by free radicals (harmful, negatively charged molecules). Few medical doctors know about oxidative stress testing, but I recommend it for patients with diabetes because they have high levels of oxidative stress, which accelerates the disease's progression. The markers of free radical activity can be measured by blood or urine tests. Elevated levels mean that the antioxidants that are normally produced in the body and ingested via foods and supplements are not effectively neutralizing the overabundance of free radicals. Your doctor can use Genova Diagnostics (800-522-4762, *www.gdx.net*) or Metametrix (800-221-4640, *www.metametrix. com*) for the test. It costs about $100, but most health insurers will cover it. People with diabetes should receive this test every six months until their values are normal.

•**Cardiovascular markers.** People with diabetes are more susceptible to heart disease. That's because elevated glucose levels accelerate the buildup of plaque in the arteries. For this reason, I recommend blood tests for homocysteine, *C-reactive protein, fibrinogen, lipoprotein a, apolipoprotein a and b* and iron. Abnormal levels of these markers are linked to the development of heart disease. I recommend a baseline test and yearly follow-up testing for people who have abnormal readings for any of these markers. Most health insurers will cover the costs of these tests.

THE SUGAR CONNECTION

Everyone knows that people who have diabetes or who are at risk for it should pay close attention to their diet. However, I'm convinced that few people realize just how damaging certain foods can be.

For example, about 20% of the average American's energy intake comes from foods such as burgers, pizza, chips, pastries and soft drinks. A 2004 study in the *American Journal of Clinical Nutrition* found that between 1980 and 1997, the average American's daily calorie consumption increased by 500 calories. Eighty percent of this increase was due to increases in carbohydrates, which include almost all sweet and starchy foods. During the same period, the prevalence of type 2 diabetes increased by 47% and the prevalence of obesity increased by 80%.

One of the worst culprits in the war on diabetes is the simple sugar fructose, which is naturally found in fruit and honey. Table sugar is half fructose (the other half is glucose, which is chemically the same as blood glucose). A type of fructose known as high-fructose corn syrup (HFCS) is especially harmful because it worsens insulin resistance. It has become the sweetener of choice for many soft drinks, ice creams, baked goods, candies/sweets, jams, yogurts and other sweetened products.

My recommendation is to put a strict limit on your consumption of foods that contain HFCS. This can be done by reducing your intake of packaged, processed foods, avoiding drinks that are high in fructose and eating as many fresh foods as possible. (Natural sources of fructose, such as fruit and honey, can be safely consumed in moderation.)

There is one exception—some liquid nutritional supplements, such as liquid vitamin formulas, contain crystalline fructose, a natural sweetener that is far less processed than HFCS and is not believed to cause dramatic increases in insulin levels.

SYMPTOMS OF DIABETES

•**Increased thirst**

•**Frequent urination** (especially at night)

•**Unexplained increase in appetite**

•**Fatigue**

•**Erection problems**

•**Blurred vision**

•**Tingling or numbness in the hands and/ or feet.**

Test for Diabetes

You have diabetes if any one of the following test results occurs on at least two different days...

●**A fasting blood glucose level of 126 mg/dL or higher.**

●**A two-hour oral glucose tolerance test** result of 200 mg/dL or higher.

●**Symptoms of diabetes combined with a random (nonfasting) blood glucose test** of 200 mg/dL or higher.

American Diabetes Association.

Tired? Moody? Adrenal Fatigue May Be to Blame

The epidemic of exhaustion affecting so many Americans today may have at its root a condition that is common and easy to correct—yet that condition often goes unrecognized by medical doctors. The culprit is adrenal fatigue (AF).

Adrenal glands produce stress hormones in response to stressful situations. With AF, the hormone response mechanism is so overwhelmed that it becomes ineffective. AF is usually triggered by long periods of mental, emotional or physical stress, and it is worsened by poor nutrition and unhealthful lifestyle choices.

In my estimation, 20% of Americans suffer from some degree of AF. And I find that this disorder often causes—or contributes to—the development of numerous other illnesses, particularly chronic fatigue syndrome and diabetes. When AF is correctly diagnosed and treated, the other conditions often are relieved as well.

STRESS HORMONE FACTORY

Located on top of each kidney is a crescent-shaped adrenal gland. The hormones these glands secrete affect blood pressure, heart rate, metabolism, liver function, immunity and the body's response to stress. Although the adrenal glands produce many hormones, two in particular

become depleted in cases of AF—*dehydroepi-androsterone* (DHEA) and *cortisol*.

●**DHEA.** The body converts DHEA into estrogen and testosterone. Abnormally low DHEA levels may contribute to cardiovascular disease, autoimmune disorders, poor resistance to infection, diabetes, weight gain, osteoporosis, sexual dysfunction, menopausal symptoms and mood disorders. DHEA also plays a role in aging. On average, the citizens of the Japanese Island of Okinawa (one of the world's longest-living people) have much higher DHEA levels at age 70 than Americans do—30% higher for men and 172% higher for women.

●**Cortisol** plays an important role in fighting infection...stabilizing blood sugar...controlling the body's use of proteins, carbohydrates and fats...and regulating the sleep cycle. Cortisol is secreted at higher levels during the fight-or-flight response to stress, providing a burst of energy, heightened alertness and decreased pain sensitivity. But when cortisol levels are elevated for long periods, production by the adrenal glands drops. Insufficient cortisol can make you prone to fatigue, infection, allergies, diabetes and thyroid dysfunction.

Depletion of DHEA and cortisol adversely affects the way your body handles stress, inflammation, blood sugar regulation, energy production, immune response and cognitive function. That's why AF can be a contributing factor in a surprising number of ailments (see "Conditions Associated with Adrenal Fatigue" on page 151). A weakened immune response plays a part in cancer as well as in recurring infections, particularly of the respiratory tract. And poor regulation of blood sugar can contribute to both diabetes and alcoholism (alcoholics often crave simple sugars, which are found in alcohol, so improving blood sugar balance can help reduce alcohol cravings).

MAKING THE DIAGNOSIS

Conventional medical doctors often don't recognize AF—even though the condition was described in medical literature in the early 20th century. It was known then as *hypoadrenia*, which means low- or under-functioning adrenal glands.

If you show signs of AF (see "Adrenal Fatigue Symptoms"), your best bet for diagnosis and

149

treatment is to see a holistic doctor. For a referral, consult the American College for Advancement in Medicine (800-532-3688, *www.acamnet. org*). *In addition to assessing your symptoms, the doctor may perform...*

•**Saliva testing to measure cortisol levels.** This test is more accurate than a blood test. A pattern of low cortisol levels throughout the day indicates AF. I ask patients to collect saliva samples in test tubes upon waking...before lunch... in the late afternoon...and before bed. Cortisol levels are normally highest in the morning and decrease throughout the day. People with severe AF usually have below-normal cortisol readings during at least two of the four time periods. I also use a saliva test that measures the DHEA level in the morning, when it is normally highest.

Saliva testing of cortisol levels is used by many research institutions, particularly to assess the effects of stress. Several commercial labs offer saliva hormone testing—including Quest Diagnostics, the nation's largest conventional medical lab, which is used by medical and naturopathic doctors. To use Quest, you must have a prescription for the test from a doctor. A lab I have used for years that usually doesn't require a doctor's order is ZRT in Beaverton, Oregon (866-600-1636, *www.salivatest.com*). The adrenal function test, including four cortisol samples and a morning DHEA reading, costs $150, which is not covered by insurance. If your state does not allow residents to order lab testing directly (check the list on the ZRT Web site), you can order the kits at the same price through my clinic (call 858-450-7120).

•**Blood pressure measurements,** taken three times—first while you lie on your back, then when you sit upright and again when you stand up. Normally, systolic (top number) and diastolic (bottom number) blood pressure will increase between 5 mm Hg and 10 mm Hg from the first reading to the third. If blood pressure *drops*, it may indicate AF—the adrenal glands may not be producing the stress hormones needed to maintain blood pressure.

•**Pupil testing,** performed in a darkened room. A practitioner shines a flashlight from the side across one eye, and the pupil should continue to get smaller. With AF, the pupil first contracts and then dilates again.

HEALING STRATEGIES

Lifestyle changes and treatment reduce symptoms in most people with AF in four to six weeks. In severe cases, full recovery may take several months. *My advice...*

•**Curb stress.** A hectic lifestyle sets the stage for AF. Are you working too hard? Is your job emotionally draining? Are your relationships unsatisfying? Try to alleviate stress and seek out emotional support.

•**Get enough rest.** Go to bed by 10 pm, and aim for eight to nine hours of sleep nightly. Whenever possible, take a 15- to 30-minute nap after lunch, even if you're getting the required amount of sleep. On weekends, nap for an hour or two.

If you have insomnia, it's vital that your sleep problems be resolved. Take a walk in the early evening or listen to relaxing music. One hour before bedtime, take 100 mg to 200 mg of *5-hydroxytryptophan* (5-HTP), an amino acid that increases brain serotonin levels and promotes relaxation...or take 0.5 mg to 3 mg of melatonin, a hormone that induces sleep. Both are available at health-food stores.

•**Eat right.** People with AF are prone to blood sugar swings that sap energy, so it is imperative to eat breakfast. I also recommend between-meal snacks, such as whole-grain toast or whey protein drinks. My favorite is Jay Robb's Whey Protein, which is naturally sweetened. It is available at major health-food stores and at *www.jayrobb. com* (877-529-7622). Almonds, walnuts and macadamia nuts are good snack foods, since they provide protein for blood sugar stabilization. Avoid simple sugars, such as those found in fruit juice and soda, as well as processed grains, such as white breads and pastas. These trigger a quick spike and subsequent drop in blood sugar levels.

Don't severely restrict salt intake unless you have high blood pressure. People with AF often benefit from salt because it helps maintain blood volume and proper circulation. Aim for 2,400 mg of sodium daily. Limit caffeinated beverages, such as coffee, tea and cola, to one cup daily because caffeine stimulates the already overtaxed adrenal glands. Avoid alcohol, which contains simple sugars.

•**Exercise in moderation.** Too little exercise is harmful, since exercise helps balance stress hormones. But overexercising worsens fatigue.

General guideline: If you're exhausted after your workout or feel more worn out than usual the next day, you're doing too much. Start by walking 15 minutes daily. As your adrenal glands recover, you can gradually increase to 45 minutes of moderately intense exercise daily.

•**Avoid lung irritants.** Cigarette smoke, air pollution and allergens can worsen AF by stimulating cortisol release. If you smoke, please quit. Avoid secondhand smoke, and reduce exposure to allergy triggers with a high-efficiency particulate air (HEPA) filter.

Clear up infections. Acute and chronic respiratory infections as well as other types of infections can exacerbate AF symptoms. To speed recovery, work with a holistic doctor, who can recommend natural immune boosters, such as the herb astralgalus.

HELPFUL SUPPLEMENTS

The following nutritional supplements are invaluable in promoting adrenal function. Take them until you recover. All are available at health-food stores. (Do not use if you are pregnant or breastfeeding.)

•**Adrenal glandular extract (AGE)** is made from cow or sheep adrenal tissue. It contains growth factors (substances that promote cell healing and regeneration) and nutrients that support gland function and adrenal repair. Take one to two tablets, two to three times daily, on an empty stomach. If you get a headache, have insomnia or feel jittery, lower the dosage.

•**Ashwagandha** is an herb used traditionally in Ayurvedic medicine for normalizing adrenal gland function. I like Jarrow's Sensoril Ashwagandha, which uses a form of the herb that has been well studied and standardized. Take one to two capsules of this product daily on an empty stomach. Side effects are rare.

•**Rhodiola rosea,** an herb that has been extensively researched, supports normal adrenal function. I recommend using a product such as Paradise Herbs' Dual Action Rhodiola, which is standardized to 3% to 5% rosavins (the active ingredient). Take 500 mg twice daily, on an empty stomach. If you feel jittery, try a lower dose.

•**B vitamins** are involved in the production of stress hormones. Particularly important is *pantothenic acid* (vitamin B-5), which is best taken at a dosage of 500 mg, three times daily. Side effects are uncommon. The rest of the B vitamins can be taken as part of a multivitamin formula.

•**Vitamin C** is needed for the adrenal glands to synthesize hormones. I recommend 1,000 mg to 2,000 mg twice daily. Reduce the dosage if you develop loose stools.

For severe cases of AF, hormone support with DHEA and cortisol may be required. This therapy should be administered by a knowledgeable doctor. The goal is to reduce the workload of the adrenal glands so they can heal. Over time, the hormone replacement can be reduced, then discontinued once the adrenals are functioning optimally.

For more information on AF, I recommend the book *Adrenal Fatigue: The 21st Century Stress Syndrome* by James Wilson, ND (Smart Publications).

ADRENAL FATIGUE SYMPTOMS

Patients with AF typically experience low energy or exhaustion (even after a good night's sleep), plus one or more of the following...

•**Light-headedness upon standing up**

•**Mood swings, especially irritability**

•**Decreased ability to cope with stress**

•**Low libido**

•**Poor concentration**

•**Impaired memory**

•**Slow recovery from illness**

•**Low back pain**

•**Salt and/or sugar cravings**

•**Inability to lose or gain weight,** despite calorie reduction or increase

CONDITIONS ASSOCIATED WITH ADRENAL FATIGUE

Although AF is not the direct cause of all the conditions below, it can be a contributing factor in...

•**Alcoholism**

•**Arthritis**

•**Asthma**

•**Exercise burnout** (becoming ill after intense workouts)

151

- **Autoimmune disorders,** such as lupus and multiple sclerosis
  - **Cardiovascular disease**
  - **Chronic fatigue syndrome**
  - **Depression and/or anxiety**
  - **Diabetes or hypoglycemia** (low blood sugar)
  - **Insomnia**
  - **Menopausal symptoms**
  - **Osteoporosis**
  - **Recurring infections**

Working Out? Drink Up

As the weather grows warmer, you may ramp up your workouts. That's great, but don't get dehydrated. Your body can lose a lot of fluid—equal to 2% or more of your body weight—from perspiring and panting. Dehydration can cause mental confusion, muscle weakness and fainting.

By the time you feel thirsty, you already may be low on fluids. A better indication of hydration level is to weigh yourself before and after exercising. A vigorous workout may trigger a loss of one to two pounds—and each pound lost should be replaced immediately by drinking 16 ounces of water.

Another indicator of hydration level is urine color. When urine looks like apple juice, you're dehydrated—so drink up until urine is pale yellow.

Also, test your *skin turgor.* Pinch the skin on the back of your hand so it tents up. If it sags slowly back into position instead of springing back quickly, you are dehydrated.

Recommended: Drink 16 ounces of water two hours before exercise…four ounces every 15 to 20 minutes during exercise…and eight to 16 ounces right after your workout. If you exercise for more than 60 minutes at a stretch, especially outside, drink a sports beverage after your workout—its carbohydrates and proteins boost energy levels, while its potassium and sodium replace electrolytes and prevent muscle cramps. Skip caffeine, which acts as a diuretic. Instead, add 5 g of *ribose* (available in powder form from health-food stores) to water or a sports drink. The body uses this naturally occurring sugar to create *adenine triphosphate* (ATP), the main energy source for all our cells. Ribose is safe for everyone and provides a welcome energy boost during and after exercise.

Noisy Knuckles and Joints

I sometimes hear from patients who complain about loose joints that crack loudly. Joints that crack usually are not painful but can cause embarrassment—during a business meeting, for example. Joint fluid contains oxygen, nitrogen and carbon dioxide gases, which are released rapidly when the joint is stretched, resulting in a pop. Your ligaments may have gotten too lax, so the bones aren't held together tightly. My patients have noticed great improvement using the homeopathic remedy *Calcarea fluorica* (at health-food stores), which provides calcium fluoride (at nontoxic levels) to tighten ligaments. Select a brand labeled "6X potency." Dissolve five tablets in your mouth, three times daily, for eight weeks or until popping subsides.

Another cause of joint cracking is dehydration of the *cartilage* (tough, elastic tissue that covers the ends of bones)—so bones no longer slide over one another smoothly and silently. To increase lubrication, take daily fish-oil supplements (do not use if you take a blood-thinning drug). Choose a product with a combined total of 1,000 mg of *eicosapentaenoic acid* (EPA) and *docosahexaenoic acid* (DHA). Within two months, this should rehydrate your joints, minimizing the snap, crackle and pop.

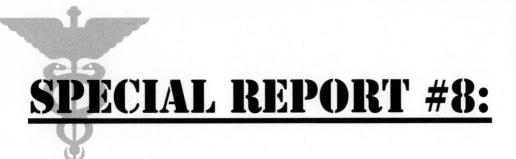

SPECIAL REPORT #8:

No-Willpower
Weight Loss

No-Willpower Weight Loss

Can Fasting Improve My Energy Levels?

Fasting can be an effective way to detoxify the body and subsequently improve energy levels. It works by giving the organs and cells of the body a rest from some of the metabolic functions they perform every second of the day. This rest allows the body to expel toxins and cleanse the tissues.

During the first day of a fast, the body burns stored sugar, known as *glycogen*. The cells also begin to burn fat for fuel, while the brain continues to burn glucose (blood sugar). During the second day of a fast, muscle tissue may be broken down into amino acids, which then are converted by the liver into glucose to feed the brain. On the third day, the fasting body goes into ketosis. During this state, the liver converts stored fat into chemicals called *ketones,* which can be used by the brain and muscles, including the heart, to sustain energy levels.

Around the third day of the fast, most people lose their hunger pains and notice increased energy and a heightened sense of awareness and clarity of mind. People may lose up to two pounds per day during this stage.

There are many different types of fasts. A water-only fast (80 ounces of water daily for one to three days) is the most aggressive type and should be used only by those in good health.

Juice fasts (80 to 100 ounces of juice daily for two to five days) also are common and are especially useful for boosting energy. These fasts often include the fresh juice of carrots, lemons, apples, beets and celery. Wheatgrass juice, which helps detoxify the liver and kidneys, and other greens also can be added.

For a modified type of fast, you can eat homemade broths and soups (three to four bowls a

Mark A. Stengler, ND, naturopathic physician in private practice, La Jolla, California...adjunct associate clinical professor at the National College of Natural Medicine, Portland, Oregon...author of many books, including *The Natural Physician's Healing Therapies* and coauthor of *Prescription for Natural Cures* (both from Bottom Line Books)...and author of the *Bottom Line/Natural Healing* newsletter.

day containing carrots, celery, chicken broth, potatoes and spices)...or drink 30 to 40 ounces
daily of detoxification meal-replacement drinks
(containing rice or pea-protein, added vitamins
and minerals and detoxifying herbs, such as milk
thistle and green tea extract), plus 32 ounces of
water. Meal-replacement drinks are commonly
available through natural health-care practitioners and at health-food stores.

People with diabetes should avoid fasts. If you
have a chronic health condition, you should fast
only under the supervision of a medical professional. People who do not react well to fasts often do better on the modified versions, such as
the use of meal-replacement drinks. If you have
little experience with fasting, work with a nutrition-oriented doctor for guidance.

Caralluma for Weight Loss

Legend has it that hunting tribes of Western India chewed the edible *Caralluma*
cactus to suppress hunger and thirst when
on long hunts. Today, Caralluma extract is being marketed as a weight-loss product that suppresses appetite and enhances metabolism.

For centuries, *Caralluma fimbriata,* the most
common form, which grows in Africa, the Ca-
nary Islands, Arabia, southern Europe, Sri Lan-
ka, Afghanistan and India, has been a normal
part of the daily diet in India. It is commonly
found growing wild in urban centers, as roadside shrubs and as boundary markers in gardens.
It can be eaten in several forms—raw, cooked as
a regular vegetable or used in preserves, such as
chutney. There have been no reports of adverse
side effects over centuries of use.

Two recent studies investigated a concentrated extract of Caralluma known as *Slimaluma.* In
the first—a randomized, double-blind, placebo-
controlled study—25 overweight or obese participants received 500 mg of Caralluma twice a
day (a dosage that is equivalent to the traditional
Indian intake of 100 grams of raw cactus) and
another 25 participants received a placebo for
eight weeks. No other changes were made in the
study participants' diets, and all were advised to

walk 30 minutes every morning and 30 minutes
every evening.

There was slightly greater average weight loss
in the Caralluma group (1.94 pounds) than in the
placebo group (1.12 pounds). More impressive
was the decrease in waist circumference—an average loss of 2.75 inches in the participants taking Caralluma, versus 1.29 inches in those taking
the placebo.

Also, researchers found that there was a statistically significant decrease in body fat, blood
pressure and hunger in members of the Caralluma group but not in the placebo group.

The second study consisted of 19 overweight
patients who were given 500-mg capsules of
Slimaluma twice daily—once before breakfast
and once before dinner—and seven patients taking a placebo for one month. More than 60% of
those taking the cactus extract lost six pounds
or more in the month. Three of the seven participants in the placebo group lost an average
of one pound...the other four gained weight or
stayed the same.

I spoke with Ronald Lawrence, MD, PhD,
a former assistant clinical professor at UCLA
School of Medicine, who reviewed the research
on Slimaluma and has recommended the extract
to many patients. He told me that most patients
lose two pounds per week for the first one to
two months of use, with no side effects, and
most report an increase in energy.

We don't know exactly how Caralluma suppresses appetite and stimulates weight loss. Researchers theorize that substances in Caralluma
known as *pregnane glycosides* prevent fat accumulation by blocking *citrate lyase,* an enzyme involved in fat formation. Pregnane glycosides also
may inhibit the hunger mechanisms in the brain.

I believe that Caralluma fimbriata will become
popular in the US because it is one of the few
weight-loss supplements that has sound clinical
data demonstrating its effectiveness.

Several companies offer the Slimaluma extract,
including Country Life (800-645-5768, *www.coun
try-life.com*), which sells a product known as
Genaslim.

Cost: $13 to $30 for one month's supply.
The recommended dosage of Slimaluma is 500
mg twice a day—30 to 45 minutes before breakfast and 30 to 60 minutes before dinner.

As with all supplements, pregnant or nursing mothers and children should use this only under a doctor's supervision.

The Hormone That May Help You Decrease Belly Fat

Dennis T. Villareal, MD, assistant professor, division of geriatrics and nutritional science, Washington University School of Medicine, St. Louis...Roberta Anding, RD, clinical dietitian, Texas Children's Hospital, Houston...*Journal of the American Medical Association.*

Researchers say an over-the-counter hormone supplement, *dehydroepiandrosterone* (DHEA), might help seniors shed stubborn belly fat. Preliminary evidence also suggests that increased levels of this natural hormone secreted by the adrenal gland might help older people avoid diabetes.

THE STUDY

Belly fat tends to accumulate with aging, just as DHEA levels begin to fall. "DHEA declines progressively with age," explains Dennis T. Villareal, MD, assistant professor of geriatrics and nutritional science at Washington University School of Medicine in St. Louis. "When we're 70 years old, we only have about 20% of the DHEA we had when we were young." From animal studies conducted in their lab, he and co-researcher Dr. John O. Holloszy suspected that falling DHEA levels might encourage weight gain. So in a double-blind trial, they had 56 non-exercising, elderly individuals take either a daily 50 milligram (mg) DHEA supplement or a placebo for six months.

RESULTS

"The replacement of DHEA, at doses of 50 mg per day, brought back DHEA levels in older persons to the range seen in youth. This resulted in a reduction in abdominal fat that was accompanied by an improvement in insulin action," says Villareal.

Participants taking the hormone supplements lost an average of 6% in visceral abdominal fat—fat deposits lying deep within the abdomen. "It averaged about one kilogram (2.2 pounds) of weight loss per person," Villareal says. Those on the placebo experienced no significant weight loss.

Patients taking the supplements also made significant improvements in insulin activity, lowering their risk for developing diabetes. That's not surprising, according to Villareal, since fatty acids released from abdominal fat cells are known to have a negative affect on insulin action. In terms of health, "what's important is that we saw a specific reduction in abdominal fat, rather than just overall weight loss," he says.

IMPLICATIONS

Villareal stresses that it's still much too early to recommend DHEA as a weight-loss supplement. "This is only a preliminary study, and we should wait for the results of large-scale, longer studies," he says. "The risks of DHEA haven't been fully defined in this short-term, relatively small study." A larger, five-year trial, involving 176 subjects, is currently under way, he says.

Roberta Anding, a clinical dietitian at Texas Children's Hospital in Houston and a spokeswoman for the American Dietetic Association, calls the findings "exciting," adding that they "open up another avenue for the management of obesity."

However, she says the supplements industry remains largely unregulated. "For the consumer, it's 'buyer beware' out there. I don't know that you can necessarily get high-quality DHEA in every health-food store, that they are all created equal."

She adds that DHEA supplements might be harmful for people with a history of hormone-sensitive cancers, such as tumors of the breast or prostate. Anding says participants in a St. Louis study who took DHEA supplements experienced a "significant" rise in blood levels of estradiol (an estrogen-like hormone) and testosterone, hormones commonly connected to breast and prostate cancers, respectively.

BOTTOM LINE

Long-term safety data holds the answer to the widespread use of DHEA. "There are going to be some people—individuals with estrogen-sensitive breast cancer or individuals who may have prostate cancer—who really should not take DHEA," Anding says.

A Natural Alternative To Sugar

Artificial sweeteners and the chemical processes used to create them have been making headlines recently. The controversy focuses primarily on the fact that the sugar in Splenda is converted to a sweetener using chlorine. Little information has been published about all the truly natural alternatives to sugar.

The result is that most Americans remain unfamiliar with healthy, natural options like Luo Han Guo, also referred to as Lo Han. A rare fruit found in China, Luo Han yields a powder 250 to 300 times sweeter than sugar.

And that's just the tip of the iceberg when it comes to the benefits of Luo Han.

As a sweetener, Luo Han Guo has no calories, does not elevate blood sugar, and is heat stable —which means it can be added to both hot and cold foods. It also helps prevent cavities and has no after-taste. These attributes make it an ideal, versatile option as a natural sweetener for tea, coffee or other beverages, and for use in making desserts.

ITS ORIGINS

While Westerners may have much to learn about Luo Han, the fruit has been used in a variety of ways, for thousands of years in China. The Lo Han Guo is a round, green perennial vine fruit in the melon family that grows wild throughout the mountainous terrain of Southwest China. Historic Chinese writings describe Song Dynasty monks brewing the fruit for medicinal beverages more than 800 years ago.

Luo Han, which is typically dried and sold in Chinese medicinal herb shops, has long been used in China and other Asian countries as a food and beverage, and also treats colds, coughs, sore throats, stomach distress, heat stroke, constipation and diarrhea.

The dried fruit is sold in a variety of forms, including whole, liquid, powdered or in a tea.

Often, in Chinese households, Luo Han is cooked with pork as a remedy for lung congestion. In fact, the *Encyclopedia of Traditional Chinese Medicine* recommends 10–15 grams—or one fruit—boiled in water per day, to address lung complaints, as Luo Han is a natural expectorant and helps clear the lungs of airborne pollutants.

The move toward using Luo Han as a sweetening agent is a more recent development.

THE VERSATILITY OF LUO HAN

In 1995, Procter & Gamble Company patented a process for making a sweetener from the fruit. Now, many sugar substitutes derived from Luo Han are available for manufacturing and personal consumption.

The Luo Han fruit, which is sold mostly in Chinese grocery stores in the United States, can be simmered into a thick, sweet juice and used during food preparation.

There are many benefits to using the Luo Han extract as a sweetening agent and sugar substitute —chief among them is the fact that the fruit contains sweet compounds called *glycosides,* specifically triterpene glycosides. The body does not break glycosides down like other simple sugars, which means blood glucose or insulin levels do not rise like they do with other sugars—making it ideal for diabetics.

Luo Han also contains high amounts of amino acids, vitamins, minerals and potent antioxidant properties, which benefit immune function and the body's ability to maintain healthy balance.

Supplements That Suppress Appetite... Really!

It's obvious that Americans are in a ferocious battle with obesity. Statistics tell us that approximately 70% of the American adult population is overweight. Unfortunately, few people realize that many over-the-counter (OTC) and prescription weight-loss medications are not very effective—and that some actually can be dangerous.

When patients come to see me for guidance in achieving healthful, permanent weight loss, I approach their needs on many levels, including their diet, level of physical activity, emotional state, hormone levels and other factors that affect body weight.

There is one area in which I (and other knowledgeable natural practitioners) can add a unique weapon in the fight against excess body weight—the use of specific nutritional supplements. Plant and other natural substances in supplement form can be used to reduce a person's appetite.

I also often can help reduce a patient's food cravings and accelerate metabolism with a selection of nontoxic dietary supplements. Contrary to what most conventional doctors will tell you, there are safe dietary supplements that work in the battle against the bulge.

NO MORE OVEREATING

It doesn't take a medical degree to know that one powerful way to lose weight successfully is to eat less—but that is much easier said than done. That's why appetite suppressants are very useful—even vital—for people who have trouble reducing their caloric intake.

Reasons for overeating vary. Some people grew up in families where portions were lavish and additional helpings were encouraged. For others, there seems to be an imbalance in the appetite control mechanism, whereby the brain does not reach a state of satiety (feeling satisfied) with normal caloric intake. A complex feedback mechanism between hormones released in the digestive tract and the brain controls this sensation of satiety.

While there's no magic bullet, I have found that the following supplements do help my patients, and there's good scientific data to back up their effectiveness and safety.

Begin by trying the first supplement. If it doesn't help within four to six weeks, then try the supplements that follow one at a time. Don't take more than one weight-loss supplement at a time.

•**Caralluma fimbriata.** This roadside shrub is found throughout many parts of India, where for centuries the whole plant has been boiled like a vegetable or eaten raw in chunks. It has an interesting history as a food to suppress hunger and thirst. During long journeys, tribesmen would pack Caralluma to help sustain themselves. Today, Caralluma is listed as a vegetable and "famine food" (a plant that is normally not used as a food crop but is consumed in times of scarcity) in the Indian Health Ministry's compilation of medicinal plants.

Gencor Pacific, an Indian herbal product provider, has done a great deal of research on this plant. It has developed Caralluma farms in India as well as a special extraction technique that can produce a therapeutic amount of this plant in capsule form. The extract is known commercially as *Slimaluma*. (For more information on Caralluma and Slimaluma, see page 156.)

I have recommended Slimaluma for many patients. In the informal trial I conducted at my clinic, 80% of users experienced reduced appetite. As in the formal research, I have found that side effects are rare. Occasionally, a person will notice minor digestive upset that usually goes away when the supplement is taken with food. Caralluma does not have a stimulant effect, as do many OTC and prescription weight-loss medications. This supplement should not be used during pregnancy or by nursing mothers. Use by children should be supervised by a doctor.

The brand I recommend is Genaslim (800-645-5768, *www.country-life.com*).

Cost: $22.99 for 60 capsules.

•**Pinolenic acid.** One new dietary supplement used to suppress appetite—without acting as a stimulant—is *pinolenic acid,* an extract from the Korean pine nut.

At a recent meeting of the American Chemical Society, scientists reported the results of a study that assessed pinolenic acid's effects on hunger and satiety. In this randomized, double-blind, placebo-controlled trial, 18 overweight women were given 3 g of pinolenic acid or a placebo (olive oil) right before eating a breakfast consisting of a moderate portion of carbohydrates.

Researchers measured blood levels of hormones associated with hunger and satiety before the supplement was taken and at regular intervals for four hours thereafter. At each interval, participants reported how hungry they felt. The pinolenic acid group reported significantly less hunger than the placebo group, rating their "desire to eat" 29% lower and their planned food intake 36% lower.

The blood tests also were revealing. After four hours, the hormones *cholecystokinin* (CCK) and *glucagon-like peptide-1* (GLP-1), produced in the small intestine, were considerably higher in the pinolenic acid group than in the placebo group. It's known that upon the consumption of food, these hormones signal satiety to the brain—so it's no surprise that the pinolenic acid group felt less hungry.

A high-quality form of pinolenic acid is available from Life Extension Foundation (800-544-4440, *www.lef.org*). The recommended dose is three 3,000-mg capsules taken 30 to 60 minutes before your highest-calorie meal of the day. Side effects are rare, but pinolenic acid is not approved for use by pregnant women or nursing mothers and should be used by children only under a doctor's supervision. A one-month supply costs $28.

•**Hydroxycitric acid (HCA).** This supplement is a compound found in the rind of a Southeast Asian fruit called *Garcinia cambogia*. The fruit is about the size of an orange and is used as a condiment in Thai and Indian cuisine. It is not a citrus fruit, but the chemical structure of HCA is similar to that of the citric acid found in citrus fruits.

Animal research has shown that HCA suppresses appetite and induces weight loss. However, results of human studies with HCA have been mixed. A study published in the *International Journal of Obesity* looked at the effect of HCA on caloric intake and satiety in overweight women and men. Twelve women and 12 men consumed a placebo—100 milliliters (ml) of tomato juice (about 3.5 fluid ounces)—three times daily for two weeks, then returned to their normal diet for two weeks and, in a final two-week phase, consumed 100 ml of tomato juice that contained 300 mg of HCA three times daily. Researchers found that participants consumed 15% to 30% fewer calories daily during the final phase than they had during the placebo phase. Other studies have not found a similar benefit.

Even though study results on HCA are not conclusive, many of my patients have benefited from this inexpensive and safe supplement. The recommended dose is 500 mg taken three times daily, just before meals. Side effects, including digestive upset, are rare. HCA should not be used by pregnant women, nursing mothers or children. It is available at many health-food stores for about $15 for a one-month supply.

•**Fiber.** One of the simplest and least expensive ways to decrease your appetite is to increase the amount of fiber in your diet. This isn't high

tech—but fiber really works, because it makes you feel full. I recommend that all of my overweight patients (regardless of whether or not they are taking a dietary supplement) include a good source of fiber in every meal. Insoluble fiber, the type that is not absorbed through the digestive tract, is an excellent choice. It is found in most vegetables, especially leafy, green ones, and fruits. For an easy way to increase your intake of insoluble fiber, include a salad or a variety of vegetables with lunch and dinner.

To achieve the greatest appetite suppression, eat vegetables at the start of meals so that you begin to feel full as early as possible. Since most people are not accustomed to eating vegetables with breakfast, I advise patients to take one to two tablespoons of ground flaxseed (grind flaxseed in a coffee grinder for five seconds) or flaxmeal (preground flaxseed is available at most health-food stores). Flaxseed can be added to cereal or a yogurt-and-fruit and/or protein shake. Be sure to drink eight to 10 ounces of water after consuming flaxseed.

You also can get appetite-suppressing fiber from supplements. A good choice is psyllium seed husks. Available at health-food stores and pharmacies, psyllium is commonly used to treat constipation, as it adds bulk to stool and stimulates peristalsis (contractions) of the intestines. For appetite suppression, start with 5 g of psyllium at the beginning of each meal along with eight to 10 ounces of water. Psyllium should not be used if you have trouble swallowing, because it expands when it's wet. Fiber supplements are best taken at least two hours before or after using vitamin and mineral supplements and pharmaceutical medications, as they can impair nutrient and drug absorption.

How to Enjoy Your Vacation and Still Stay Slim

Counting calories isn't necessary. Calories are a factor in fat reduction. The higher the number of calories from food, the more energy you must expend burning them off. With my system, counting calories becomes obsolete. The real issue is focusing on quality foods in moderate portions.

If you focus on quality foods when you travel and the right ratio of the different types of foods, the calorie count will remain at a level where you can lose weight.

•**Eat smaller meals.** Eating smaller, more regular meals throughout the day helps to quell the appetite and level the blood sugar. This is a long-term strategy for fat reduction.

•**Do not skip meals.** I would say 30 percent of all my weight-loss patients tell me on our initial visit they skip breakfast. Never skip a meal, especially on the road. This is a signal to the body to conserve energy and store fat.

If time is an issue, prepare breakfast the night before your flight, or make yourself a protein shake by combining 1 scoop of soy or whey protein powder with soy or rice milk and 1 to 2 tablespoons of ground-up flaxseeds. Add some blueberries or another fruit that you like.

This takes a whopping two minutes and supplies you with protein, carbohydrates, good essential fatty acids and fiber. It will help to level out your blood sugar and prevent fat storage. It will also increase your energy and mental sharpness.

•**Harness the power of plant foods.** Don't forget the power of plant foods when you're on a fat-reduction diet. Vegetables and some fruits are excellent sources of fiber, which helps to bind fat from foods and expel it in the stool.

Fiber also helps to slow the release of sugar from foods into the bloodstream. This is especially true of soluble fiber—found in oat bran, dried beans, peas, rice bran, barley and apple skin. Make sure fresh fruit and vegetables are cleaned thoroughly, especially if traveling overseas.

Plant foods are also excellent sources of phytonutrients that aid the body in many ways, including the process of "burning fat"—that is, fat metabolism. You can get the full spectrum of amino acids from the combination of various plant foods. They are also very important for detoxification. That's significant because proper detoxification removes toxins that cause fat storage and water retention.

•**Watch your water intake.** Drinking an adequate amount of water is critical for weight loss. Dehydration, even at a marginal level, actually causes the body to store water, and water retention is a large factor in weight gain. In addition, water is essential for detoxification. Purchase bottled water if you are traveling to areas where water quality is suspect.

You should drink at least six to eight 8-ounce glasses of water daily (48 to 64 ounces). Also, avoid those substances that cause dehydration such as caffeine (coffee), salt and alcohol.

•**Identify your food sensitivities.** And be extra-cautious when you travel. One of the ways I expedite the weight-loss process for my patients is to identify their food sensitivities. Food sensitivities cause water retention and make metabolism and detoxification more sluggish.

Lose Weight with Apple Cider Vinegar

Patients often tell me that apple cider vinegar has helped them with a variety of ailments. Until recently, there was little research to back up these claims.

CURE-ALL?

Apple cider vinegar has been singled out as beneficial for a variety of conditions, including leg cramps, stomach upset, sore throat, sinus problems, high blood pressure, obesity, osteoporosis and arthritis. It also has been used to help rid the body of toxins, improve concentration, slow aging, reduce cholesterol and fight infection.

It is used topically to treat acne, sunburn, shingles and insect bites…as a skin toner…and to prevent dandruff. Many women add it to bathwater to treat vaginitis. Two of its most common uses are for weight loss and arthritis.

THE SCIENTIFIC EVIDENCE

Recent studies have found that consuming apple cider vinegar can improve insulin resistance, a condition in which muscle, fat and liver cells have become resistant to the uptake of the hormone *insulin* and the blood sugar *glucose* needed to provide fuel for energy.

This is common among people who have diabetes as well as in some people we consider prediabetic—that is, their blood glucose and insulin levels are approaching the numbers that define diabetes. People with insulin resistance are more likely to be overweight and have increased cholesterol and triglyceride levels as well as high blood pressure.

A study at the University of Arizona examined the effects of apple cider vinegar on 29 participants (10 had type 2 diabetes, 11 had signs that they could become diabetic and eight were healthy but "insulin sensitive"). All participants fasted and were randomly asked to drink either a vinegar solution (two tablespoons or 20 g of apple cider vinegar, some water and a bit of saccharin for flavor) or a placebo drink. The drinks were followed by a high-carbohydrate meal of one white bagel, butter and orange juice.

Researchers found that postmeal spikes of insulin and glucose in the vinegar group were significantly lower in those who had insulin resistance and slightly lower in those who had diabetes, compared with those in the placebo group. Other research has shown that apple cider vinegar helps control insulin and glucose spikes in healthy people.

HOW IT WORKS

Researchers theorize that the *acetic acid* in any vinegar, including apple cider vinegar, interferes with the enzymes that digest carbohydrates, so carbs pass through the digestive tract without being absorbed. Acetic acid also has been shown to affect enzymes that alter glucose metabolism in liver and muscle cells, reducing insulin spikes.

Because high levels of insulin promote inflammation, taking vinegar to maintain insulin levels will control any inflammation in the body. This may explain why vinegar eases arthritis pain.

DOSAGE

People can try apple cider vinegar for weight loss, blood sugar balance and other traditional uses, including arthritis relief. Dilute one to two tablespoons (some people use as little as two teaspoons to start with) in an equal amount of water, and drink it at the beginning of a meal.

Sometimes it is more convenient to take it in supplement form. A good product is Apple Cider Vinegar Plus, which is made by Indiana Botanic Gardens (800-644-8327, *www.botanicchoice.com*). Take three capsules a day (one with each meal).

Apple cider vinegar can cause digestive upset in some people. If you have active ulcers, use caution when taking apple cider vinegar.

SPECIAL REPORT #9:

How to Find a Good Holistic Doctor In Your Area

How to Find a
Good Holistic Doctor
In Your Area

How to Find a Good Holistic Doctor in Your Area

Finding a holistic doctor is easier than ever, but finding a good one is a different matter. When I was in college, alternative medicine was in its infancy, and naturopaths were scarce. (I had to drive three hours to the nearest one!)

Today, things are different. Alternative and complementary medicine have become big business, and many conventionally trained physicians have jumped on the bandwagon. While some of these doctors are quite good, many others have only the most basic knowledge of alternative and natural therapies—not nearly enough to treat people with chronic illnesses.

Example: A prominent hospital in the San Diego area has what they call, an "integrative center," but several of its practitioners dispense little more than multivitamins and coenzyme Q10 supplements. Many of my patients tried this center before they found me, and I wouldn't want you to get similar poor results before you find good care.

GETTING STARTED

Searching professional associations can be a good place to start because they specify which treatment modalities a particular provider offers.

Example: If you want a doctor who does nutritional therapies, homeopathy, or oxygen therapies, these membership directories will often tell you...

•**American Association of Naturopathic Physicians**—866-538-2267 or *www.naturopath ic.org*

•**International College of Integrative Medicine**—866-464-5226 or *www.icimed.com*

•**American College for Advancement in Medicine**—800-532-3688 or *www.acamnet.org*

The downside is that directories don't necessarily tell you whether the doctor is any good.

Mark A. Stengler, ND, naturopathic physician in private practice, La Jolla, California...adjunct associate clinical professor at the National College of Natural Medicine, Portland, Oregon...author of many books, including *The Natural Physician's Healing Therapies* and coauthor of *Prescription for Natural Cures* (both from Bottom Line Books)...and author of the *Bottom Line/Natural Healing* newsletter.

Membership in an association doesn't guarantee a great practitioner—only that he or she has met certain standards and pays annual dues.

WHAT HELPS

The best way to find a good holistic doctor is to talk to people who see one regularly. A great place to get recommendations is your local health food store. Ask your fellow customers and store workers about their experiences. After you've spoken to five or ten people, you'll start hearing the same one or two doctor's names that are the ones you should call.

Once you're at the doctor's office, you can gauge how good he or she is by asking the following magic question, "*What are the root causes of my condition, and how shall we address them?*" Mediocre holistic doctors will look at your symptoms and prescribe their remedies (just like conventional physicians who prescribe drugs). Superior practitioners look for the root cause of your condition to achieve true healing.

How to Find a Reputable Acupuncturist

If you are interested in trying acupuncture for low-back pain or other muscle aches, I recommend getting a referral from a local chiropractor, massage therapist or friend who has personal experience with a local acupuncturist. You also can find practitioners in your area by contacting the American Association of Acupuncture and Oriental Medicine (866-455-7999, *www.aaaomonline.org*).

Look for a practitioner who graduated from an accredited school—you can confirm his/her accreditation with the Council of Colleges of Acupuncture and Oriental Medicine (301-476-7790, *www.ccaom.org*). Make sure that he has been in practice for at least two years.

Also, be wary of medical doctors who practice acupuncture. They are not required to complete the same three- or four-year program as licensed acupuncturists.